The Grub Wrangler

Heartfelt Grapeseed Oil Recipes with Benefits

A Whiskey Salvation Cookbook

Chrissy Hartmann

The Grub Wrangler

Heartfelt Grapeseed Oil Recipes with Benefits

A Whiskey Salvation Cookbook

Chrissy Hartmann

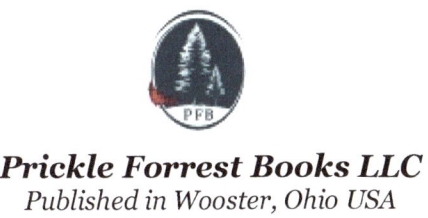

Prickle Forrest Books LLC
Published in Wooster, Ohio USA

Copyright

Publisher Information
Prickle Forrest Books LLC
prickleforrestllc@sssnet.com

First Printing

Copyright© January 2025 by Chrissy Hartmann

Cover Designer GetCovers

Book Interior Designers Christina Benchoff, Cary Harter, Cyndi Boyer, Alexandra Musselman, and Renee Mack

Editor Prickle Forrest Books

Photographer: Jacob Benchoff

Library of Congress Control Number: 2024927082
ISBN (Digital) 978-1-965780-02-2
ISBN (Paperback) 978-1-7379288-6-7

Printed in the United States of America

Author/Publisher's Note:
No part of this publication may be reproduced, stored in a retrieval system, or transmitted in any form or by any means, electronic, mechanical, photocopying, recording, scanning, or otherwise, without the prior written permission of the author/publisher, except in the case of brief quotations embodied in critical reviews and certain other noncommercial uses permitted by copyright law. For permission requests, write to the author/publisher, addressed "Attention: Permissions Coordinator," at the address below.
Prickle Forrest Books LLC
257 Winkler Drive
Wooster, OH 44691

The recipes and information in this book are provided in good faith and have been thoroughly tested and reviewed. However, the author and/or publisher are not responsible for any errors or omissions, or for any adverse effects resulting from the use of the recipes and suggestions contained herein.

The nutritional information and health benefits described in this book are based on research and literature available at the time of publication. They are not intended as medical advice. For health-related questions, please consult a healthcare professional.

Third-Party Permissions

Papa Fike's Original Seasoning
Copyright © 2023 by Papa Fike's Seasoning LLC by permission of Papa Fike's Seasoning, LLC (Adriana and Brad Fike).
https://papafikesseasoning.com

Olive Layne Oils
Copyright © 2023 by Olive Lane Oils, LLC by permission of Olive Layne Oils, LLC
https://olivelaneoils.com

Pixabay.com
Copyright © 2023 by Pixabay.com by permission of the photographers of pixabay.com.
https://pixabay.com

Papa Fike's Fiken Awesome Seasonings

Craving flavor-packed, guilt-free meals? Look no further than Papa Fike's seasoning collection. With Papa Fike's, you can enjoy the goodness of tasty food without the added sugar and MSG.

Introducing Papa Fike's Original, blackened, and salt and vinegar Blends – the ultimate all-purpose seasoning you've been waiting for! With this versatile seasonings, you can elevate the flavor of any dish without worrying about its ingredients. Whether you're cooking eggs, veggies, beef, chicken, tacos, or soups, this seasoning is your perfect companion. Say goodbye to the hassle of experimenting with different seasonings – Papa Fike's Original, blackened, and salt and vinegar Blends take care of the proportions for you. Simply flip the cap, sprinkle it on your food, and let the magic happen. No more second-guessing, just delicious meals every time. Plus, enjoy the convenience of FREE SHIPPING with every order!
https://fikebrandsllc.com/
Spice up your culinary adventures with Papa Fike's Original, BLACKENED, AND SALT AND VINEGAR blends today!

- *Filled with ingredients easily pronounced*
- *- No MSG*
- *No sugar added*
- *- No Ssalt added*

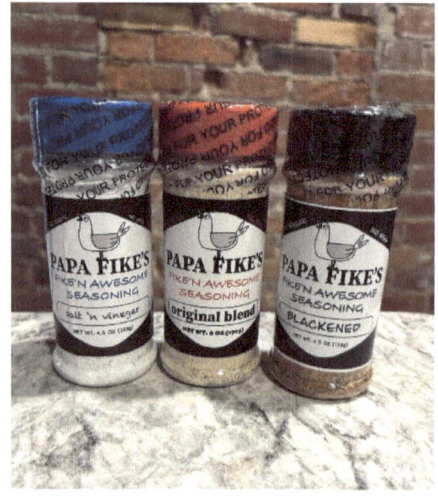

Dedication

To Paul Harvey and "The Rest of the Story"

Acknowledgements

First, I'd like to thank Paul Harvey and his radio show "And the Rest of The Story." If I hadn't heard his one program on grapeseed I would probably not be here today. So "thank you for that gold nugget of information. It's a life changer!"

Next, I'd like to thank five creatively talented people, Jacob Benchoff, Cyndi Boyer, Cary Harter, Alexandra Musselman, and Renee Mack. Five individuals who were significant with helping me make sure the book had scrumptious recipes and deliciously tempting photos of them.

I would also like to thank my family doctor, cardiologist, nutritionists, and the chefs who took the time to answer my questions with regards to grapeseed oil and cooking. Your advice has been well received and appreciated.

Big-big thanks go to the PFB Book Cover Review Team who helped critique the cover of this cookbook. Your talent in book covers is highly remarkable and is without a doubt topnotch.

Thanks also goes to Brad Fike and his daughter Adriana and their development of the Papa Fike's Seasonings. Your original, blackened, and salt and vinegar are made so deliciously yummy that they make my taste buds howl for more.

A special thanks goes to my mom, Julia Martini who first taught me to cook. Without your guidance and talent for making the simplest meals taste extraordinarily tasty I wouldn't have tied on the apron to start my own journey into cooking.

And let's not forget a special thanks to my dad, Edward Hartmann who instilled in me the tenacity to get the job done. He's the one that's always said "practice makes perfect" which pushes me to keep trying with my recipes until they make the taste buds sing.

I also want to thank my hubby, K.O. Benchoff and my son, Jacob Benchoff for continuing to believe in my writing and for being my taste testers and back-up photographers for a number of these dishes. Without question, your taste buds are truly golden and your eye for detail is spot on.

And finally, I want to thank God because without his blessings, I would not be where I am today. Thank you, Lord for providing the talent to write, cook, and for the bounty you provide for those who use this cookbook.

Love and thanks to you all!

Chrissy Hartmann

Contents

Chapter 1 Introduction 1
Chapter 2 History of Grapeseed Oil 3
_2.1 Culinary Benefits 4
_2.2 Grapeseed Oil Health Benefits 5
_2.3 Dangers of Grapeseed Oil 7
Chapter 3 The Making of Grapeseed Oil 9
_3.1 Grapeseed Oil Production 10
_3.2 Grapeseed Oil versus Grapeseed Extract 11
_3.3 The Grapes 12
_3.4 Grapeseed Production 14
_3.5 Reasons for Choosing Grapeseed Oil 15
_3.6 Grapeseed Antioxidants 16
_3.7 Grape Varieties 18
_3.8 Grapeseed Oil Nutritional Value 20
_3.9 Daily Recommended Allowances 21
_3.10 Grapeseed Oil — Safe for the Trail if Ridden Right 22
Chapter 4 Sunrise Delights 25
_4.1 Blueberry Flapjacks 26
_4.2 Healthy Morning Smoothie 28
_4.3 Western Sunrise Slices 29
_4.4 Saddle Hearty Oatmeal 30
_4.5 Western Banana-Cran Bites 32
_4.6 Cowboy Granola Crunch 33
_4.7 Texas Steak and Egg Fajita 35
_4.8 Feta Fiesta Spinach Eggs 36

Chrissy Hartmann

_4.9 Texas Sunshine Muffins 38
_4.10 Pumpkin Harvest Berry Bread 40

Chapter 5 Savory Starters 43
_5.1 Spicy Hummus with Fresh Veggies 44
_5.2 Butternut Chipotle Turkey Chili 46
_5.3 Robust Spinach Artichoke Dip 48
_5.4 Smokey Orange Cauliflower Wings 50
_5.5 Rustic Chili Potato Wedges 52
_5.6 Grilled Veggie Bob 53
_5.7 Chicken Pepper Cranberry Salad 54
_5.8 Fire Blackened Shrimp 56
_5.9 Turkey Stuffed Mushrooms 58
_5.10 Plum Delicious Fried Greenies 60
_5.11 Cauliflower Cow Patties 62
_5.12 Chipotle Chicken Wings 63

Chapter 6 Main Course Marvels 65
6.1 Blackened Catfish with Lemon Cream Sauce 66
6.2 Zesty Lemon Chicken 68
6.3 Chipotle Shrimp Scampi 69
6.4 Spirited Beef Stir-Fry 70
6.5 Woodland Mushroom Risotto 72
6.6 Pecan Berry Chicken 73
6.7 Pork Tenderloin with Apple Compote 74
6.8 Christmas Spinach Chicken 75
6.9 Rodeo Peppered Beef 76
6.10 Chipotle Steak Taco 77

6.11 Sundance Tuna Melts *78*
6.12 Rustler's Beef Stew *80*
6.13 Chicken Soft Taco *82*
6.14 Stuffed Sausage Peppers *84*
6.15 Texas-Two Step Barbecue Chicken *86*
6.16 Seared Salmon *88*
6.17 Southwest Black Bean Burger *89*
6.18 Cowboy Salad *90*
6.19 Calico Beans.. *92*

Chapter 7 Satisfying Sidekicks *95*
_7.1 Yukon Golden Roasted Potatoes *96*
_7.2 Mediterranean Lemon Salad.. *97*
_7.3 Mushroom Onion Spinach Saute *98*
_7.4 Green Bean Roundup with Bacon.. *99*
_7.5 Campfire Roasted Asparagus *100*
_7.6 Balsamic Glazed Carrots *102*
_7.7 Lonestar Tater Salad *104*
_7.8 Lemon Broccoli..105*
_7.9 Spicy Sweet Taters *106*
_7.10 Pony Up Pasta Salad..107*
_7.11 Buckshot Brussel Sprouts... *108*
_7.12 Crispy Chipotle Kale Chips..110*
_7.13 Chuckwagon Cornbread *112*
_7.14 Texas Hash... *114*

_Chapter 8 Delicious Desserts *117*
_8.1 Iowa Dusty Delights *118*
_8.2 Colorado Berry Crumble *120*

Chrissy Hartmann

_8.3 Trails End Banana Bread 122
_8.4 Apple Cinnamon Cake 124
_8.5 Cowboy Cow Chips 126
_8.6 Heavenly Berry Parfait 128
_8.7 Toasted Pecan Clusters 129
_8.8 Lemon Herding Cakes 130
_8.9 Homestead Pumpkin Funnel Cakes 132
_8.10 Peanut Brittle 134
_8.11 Texas Carrot Cake 136
_8.12 Cowboy cookies 138

_Chapter 9 Dressings, Drizzles, and more 141
_9.1 Classic Balsamic Vinaigrette 142
_9.2 Lemon-Honey Dijon Dressing 143
_9.3 Sesame Dressing: 144
_9.4 Sweet Orange Dressing 145
_9.5 Raspberry-Lime Vinaigrette 146
_9.6 Maple-Dijon Glaze 147
_9.7 Honey Mustard Glaze 148
_9.8 Sweet-N-Sour Dressing 149
_9.9 Homemade Mayonnaise 150
_9.10 Chipotle Drizzle 151
_9.11 Honey Barbecue Sauce 152
_9.12 Spicy Vidalia Sauce 153
_9.13 Lemon Cream Sauce 154
_9.14 Plum Delicious Ginger Dipping Sauce 155

Chapter 10 Cooking and Baking Tips 157

_10.1 Cooking Tips 158
_10.2 Baking Tips..159
Chapter 11 Cooking Oils.. 161
_11.1 More On Vegetable Oils 166
_11.2 Storage Life of Oils 169
_11.3 Signs of Rancid Oils.. 171
_11.4 Types of Fats Found in Cooking Oils 173
Chapter 12 Culinary Techniques 176
Chapter 13 Cooking Conversions..179
_13.1 Measurement Conversions.. 180
_13.2 Temperature Conversions 181
_13.3 Target Temperatures 182
Chapter 14 Cowboy-style Glossary 185
Dear Reader: 189
Chrissy's Other Books.. 190
About The Author... 191
Index..192

Chrissy Hartmann

Chapter 1 Introduction

Howdy, culinary trailblazers! Welcome to a cookbook that's as good for your heart as it is for your taste buds –

Time to cowboy up with ...

"The Grub Wrangler
Heartfelt Grapeseed Oil Recipes with Benefits."

Saddle up and join us on a flavorful journey through the heartland of health-conscious cooking.

Our tale begins with the legendary Paul Harvey's "Rest of the Story," echoing across the airwaves and introducing me to the wonders of grapeseed oil. This liquid gold, rich in antioxidants, became more than just a kitchen companion; it became a remedy, easing the pains of neuropathy and setting me on a path to improved health.

It all started with grapeseed extract first. I heard from Paul Harvey's show the vitamin was high in antioxidants and had some healing powers that could possibly ease the pain from neuropathy I suffered in my feet. So, I purchased a bottle or two and started taking it. After 3 months, I figured the dietary nutrient must have done some healing because the pain in my feet disappeared . I found soon after that, stores carried the grapeseed oil too. Unfortunately, I stored it away in the pantry and thought nothing of it until I hit the spry age of 43.

After a heart attack with the right coronary artery blocked in 3 different spots at 70%, 80%, and 90% , this author discovered that grapeseed oil might be the unsung hero of heart-healthy cooking. With a resolve as strong as a cowboy's grit, I've embraced this oil, witnessing not just a culinary transformation but a journey towards wellness.

Why keep such a revelation under wraps? When something does your heart and soul good, you share it with the world. Right?
Hence, this cookbook was born – a collection of recipes straight from my chuckwagon and those of my culinary compadres, celebrating the joyous marriage of flavor and health.

From dawn's first light to the starry dessert skies, this cookbook covers every course on the trail. Start your day right with breakfast recipes that'll have you rustling up energy like a ranch hand at sunrise. Wrangle appetizers that pack a punch, leaving your taste buds doing a square dance. And for the main course and sides, whether you're barbecuing chicken or roasting taters, grapeseed oil is the trusty partner that brings both flavor and heart health to the table.

Chrissy Hartmann

As the sun sets, don't forget about the sweet tooth in you, desserts crafted with the same heartiness and a touch of cowboy sweetness. And for an extra bonus, drizzle on some homemade sauces or dress your salads with concoctions that'll have you singing praises to the chuckwagon gods.

Why is grapeseed oil the John Wayne of the kitchen?

Well Partner, it's versatile. Sauteing, baking, grilling, or dressing – grapeseed oil plays nice with every dish on the roundup. With a high smoke point, it won't be kicking up a fuss, ensuring that your culinary creations are as delightful as a lullaby under the stars.

Come join the culinary journey, where the trail is paved with the golden glow of grapeseed oil and every recipe tells a tale of heartiness and happiness. So, hitch your appetite to a new kind of cowboy feast, where flavor meets health on the open range. Now some folk may wonder why they just don't use grapeseed extract instead, right? After all it's got the same health benefits, but in a highly concentrated form and it's easier to travel with.

Hey, cowboy, please do. But remember, if you cook with an oil or bake with one, why not use one that's actually heart healthy? Those other oils out there don't carry quite the same benefits grapeseed oil provides. Sure, they come close, but with its abundance of antioxidants and light flavor plus a few other benefits you can find throughout the book, why not use both then? I do. It's been ten plus years since my first ticker attack, and I've not had another since I've changed my ways. So, with a healthy diet, exercise, and a positive attitude you too can find yourself on the trail to happiness.

Saddle up to taste the beauty of grapeseed oil and let's ride together into a hart healthier sunset! So, Cowboy Up With Grapeseed Oil and enjoy the Heartfelt Healthy Recipes with Benefits!

Thanks and enjoy!

Chrissy Hartmann

Chapter 2 History of Grapeseed Oil

Shooting straight from the hip, here is the history of grapeseed oil.

Grapeseed oil comes from the seeds of grapes. It's history with cooking is somewhat short, but the oil itself is linked to biblical times dating back to the Old Testament known as Vitis vinifera when grapes were believed in the 6000-5000 BC era to have been made into wine. As the wine was made, the oil was removed from the seeds and was thought to be used as an "ancient healer."

There are some rumors out there that the Prophet Daniel may have used it when he went on a ten-day fast with his meals consisting of "Pure" and water. Now, we here at the chuckwagon have searched high and low for confirmation regarding this fact, but at the moment of publication only one reference/resource, has been located to confirm this and unfortunately it looks a bit rough around the edges. we usually prefer at least half a dozen or so, but since we had no luck, please use the biblical information mentioned here at your own discretion. If we do manage to rustle up more facts, I'll be sure as rain to update this here cookbook.

Initially, the oil was primarily a byproduct of the wine-making industry, with grape seeds considered waste. However, in the late 20th century it gained popularity due to its health benefits and culinary versatility. Grapeseed oil is often associated with the Mediterranean diet with being known for its ticker-healthy properties.

Grapeseed oil is celebrated for its various cooking and health benefits, but like most things, it too has some dangers you don't want to forget about either. So, on that note, saddle up and ride on to partner up with this here heart-healthy grapeseed oil and our recipes with benefits. Now giddy up!

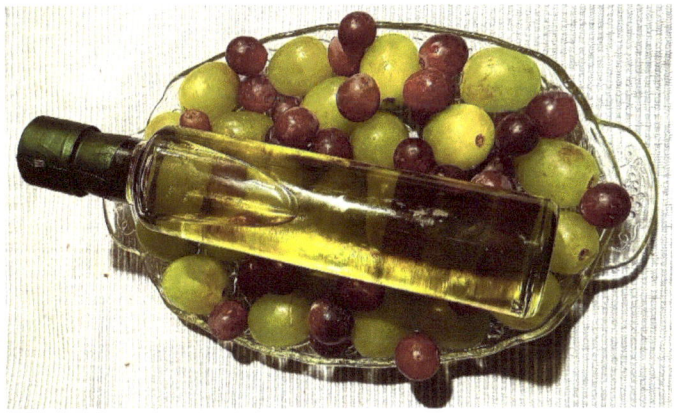

Chrissy Hartmann

2.1 Culinary Benefits

In the rugged world of cowboys, where the skillet rules the kitchen and simplicity is key, grapeseed oil emerges as a culinary ally. Extracted from the seeds of grapes brings a unique set of benefits to any cowboys cooking. With its high smoke point, light flavor profile, and healthful properties, grapeseed oil adds a touch of finesse to a cowboy's cuisine, enhancing the robust flavors of what might normally taste like trail cooking while aligning with the practical demands of life in the west.

1. high smoke point
- It is commonly used for sauteing, frying, grilling, and baking because of its high smoke point (around 420°F, which makes it suitable for high-heat cooking methods.

2. Neutral taste
- It's mild flavor complements salad dressings, allowing other ingredients' flavors to shine.

3. Baking
- Grapeseed oil can be a suitable substitute for butter or other oils in baking recipes.

4. Shelf life
- Store it in a cool, dark place, away from direct sunlight and heat, with the container tightly sealed.
- Use clean, dry utensils to avoid contamination.
- When properly stored, grapeseed oil can last up to 6-12 months unopened, and 3-6 months opened.

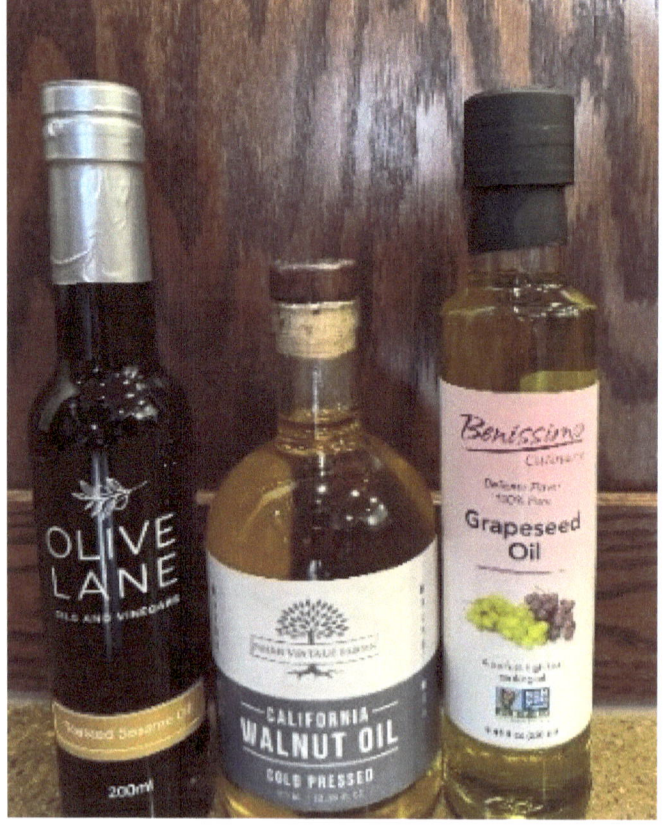

2.2 Grapeseed Oil Health Benefits

Grapeseed oil offers several potential health benefits due to its nutritional profile and unique properties. On the ranch, while our cowboys tend to the livestock and land, we here in the chuckwagon like to make sure we feed our boys with the best food even if it's only steaks and beans. They work from dawn to dusk with the work demanding and it's my job to feed them healthy good tasting meals that gives their bodies a boost and keeps the heart strong and the energy up. With the list below, you'll find some of the benefits and why you'll find no other oil inside my skillets and pots but grapeseed oil. Now cowboy up and read on!

1. Heart Health: Grapeseed oil is high in polyunsaturated fats, particularly omega-6 fatty acids, which can help reduce bad LDL cholesterol levels and improve heart health when used as part of a balanced diet.

2. Antioxidants: It contains antioxidants like vitamin E, which can help protect cells from damage caused by free radicals, potentially reducing the risk of chronic diseases and protects against tissue damage.

3. Anti-Inflammatory Properties: The presence of polyphenols in grapeseed oil may have anti-inflammatory effects, helping to reduce inflammation in the body.

4. Weight Management: Grapeseed oil is low in saturated fat and calories, making it a lighter option for cooking and contributing to weight management when used in moderation.

5. Skin Health: The antioxidants and vitamin E in grapeseed oil can be beneficial for skin health. It is commonly used in cosmetics and skincare products for its moisturizing and anti-aging properties.

6. Blood Sugar Regulation: Some studies suggest that grapeseed oil may help improve insulin sensitivity and regulate blood sugar levels, potentially benefiting individuals with diabetes *Remember always check with your doctor before making any dietary changes so not to throw off your medication routine.

7. Reduced Risk of Chronic Diseases: The antioxidants in grapeseed oil may contribute to a reduced risk of various chronic diseases, including cardiovascular diseases and some cancers.

Chrissy Hartmann

8. Digestive Health: Grapeseed oil may promote better digestion by supporting the body's ability to break down and absorb nutrients from food.

9. Lowering Blood Pressure: Some research indicates that grapeseed oil may have a mild blood pressure-lowering effect, which can be advantageous for individuals with hypertension.

* It's important to note that while grapeseed oil has potential health benefits, it should be used in moderation as part of a balanced diet. Excessive consumption of any oil can contribute to excess calorie intake, which may lead to weight gain. Additionally, individual responses to dietary components can vary, so it's essential to consult with a healthcare professional for personalized dietary advice.

* Always consult your medical posse first before changing any medications and/or adding anything new to your food or medical regimen.

2.3 Dangers of Grapeseed Oil

While grapeseed oil is generally considered safe for most cowboys and cowgirls and offers numerous benefits, there are a few potential concerns and dangers associated with its use, so take caution when using. We don't want any of this oil putting an end to all those happy trails you have yet to travel. So saddle up and read on!

1. Allergies: Some individuals may be allergic to grape products, including grapeseed oil. Allergic reactions can range from mild skin irritation to more severe symptoms like itching, swelling, hives, or anaphylaxis. If you have a known grape or grapeseed allergy, you should avoid products containing grapeseed oil.

2. High Omega-6 Fatty Acids: Grapeseed oil is relatively high in omega-6 fatty acids, and an excessive intake of omega-6 fatty acids, especially when not balanced with omega-3 fatty acids, can potentially contribute to inflammation in the body. It's important to maintain a balanced omega-6 to omega-3 ratio in your diet.

3. Not Suitable for High-Heat Cooking: While grapeseed oil has a higher smoke point than many other vegetable oils, it's not as heat-stable as some other options like coconut oil, ghee, or avocado oil. Using grapeseed oil at very high temperatures over 420°F can cause it to break down and release potentially harmful compounds.

4. Quality Concerns: The quality of grapeseed oil can vary widely. Some commercial grapeseed oils are processed with solvents and may contain impurities. It's essential to **choose cold-pressed** or **expeller-pressed**, **organic, and high-quality grapeseed oil** to ensure you're getting the full nutritional benefits without unwanted chemicals.

5. Weight Gain: While grapeseed oil is low in saturated fat, it is calorie dense. Overconsumption of any oil can contribute to excess calorie intake and potential weight gain. Moderation is key.

6. Not Suitable for All Cooking Methods: Grapeseed oil may not be the best choice for all cooking methods. It's more suitable for sautéing, stir-frying, grilling, or as a salad dressing. It may not be ideal for baking, where the texture and flavor may differ from recipes that traditionally use butter. I suggest you test it out before you serve to others.

Chrissy Hartmann

7. Dog Warning: And remember, though you might like to share a bit of your food with your best friend, grapes and that includes the grapeseed oil, raisins, and anything you might make with it is dangerous to your dog. Even , though it's beneficial for us, it's not healthy and most often fatal for your dogs. Please be careful when you eat anything made with grapes or grapeseed oil around your best friend.

* As with any dietary choice, it's important to use grapeseed oil in moderation and consider your individual health, dietary, and allergy concerns. If you have specific health conditions or dietary restrictions, consult with a healthcare professional or a registered dietitian for personalized advice on using grapeseed oil or choosing the best oil for your needs.

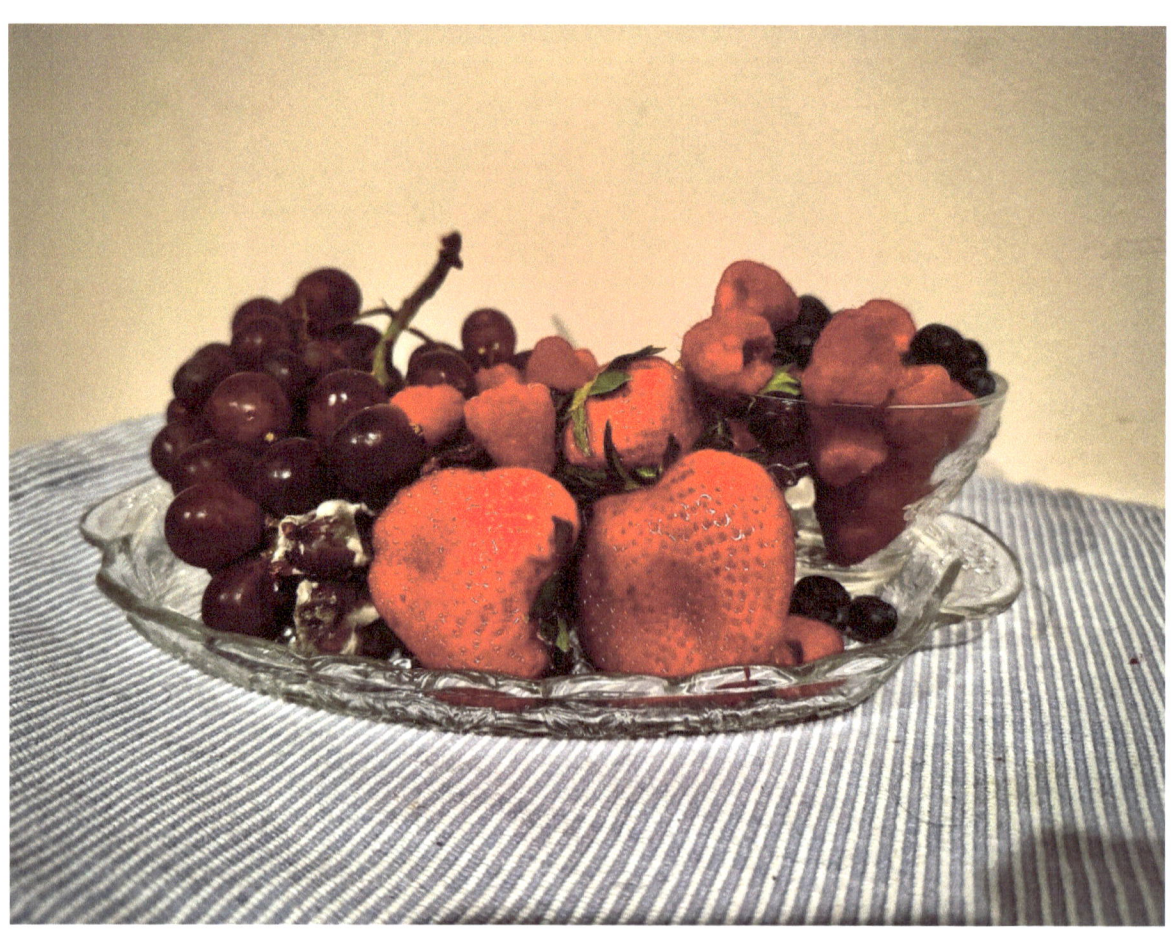

Chapter 3 The Making of Grapeseed Oil

Ever wonder what goes into the magic elixir that's been helping to keep us healthy here on the ranch?

Let me spill the beans about grapeseed oil – the unsung hero of our chuckwagon cooking.

Well, partner, it all begins in the heart of the vineyards where grape seeds are usually cast aside. These seeds find new purpose. The grapes, packed with potential undergo a meticulous process of pressing and extraction. The result "a golden hued liquid treasure" known as grapeseed oil. It's like capturing the spirit of the wild west transforming overlooked seeds into a culinary sidekick that elevates this here cowboy's cuisine. So, pull on those boots and grab your hat, let's delve into the flavorful journey of how grapeseed oil becomes the hero in these here chuckwagon adventures.

Chrissy Hartmann

3.1 Grapeseed Oil Production

1. Seed Collection: Grapes are harvested for wine production, and about 2 tons of grapes are used to make 1 liter of the yellow-green grapeseed oil. The seeds are collected as a byproduct. Grapes from wine production are often preferred, as they tend to have higher-quality seeds.

2. Cleaning: The collected grape seeds are cleaned to remove any remaining grape pulp, skins, and stems. This cleaning process ensures that the oil extraction is not compromised by impurities.

3. Drying: The cleaned grape seeds may be dried to reduce their moisture content. This step is essential because excess moisture can lead to spoilage during storage and affect the quality of the oil.

4. Cold-Pressing or Solvent Extraction:
-Cold-Pressing (Preferred Method): In this method, the dried seeds are mechanically pressed to release the oil. The pressing is typically done at low temperatures to retain the oil's flavor and nutritional qualities. Cold-pressed grapeseed oil is often considered higher quality.
- Solvent Extraction (Less Common): Some commercial operations use solvents like hexane to extract the oil from the seeds. Solvent extraction can be more efficient but may result in a lower-quality oil if not properly processed and refined.

5. Filtration: The extracted oil is then typically filtered to remove any remaining solids or impurities.

6. Refining (Optional): In some cases, grapeseed oil may undergo a refining process to remove any remaining impurities, odor, and flavor. This process may include degumming, neutralization, and deodorization.

7. Packaging: The final, refined grapeseed oil is packaged in containers, such as glass or plastic bottles or even tin cans and prepared for distribution.

It's important to note that the best grapeseed oils are often cold-pressed and minimally processed to preserve their natural flavor and nutritional benefits. Additionally, the quality of the grapes and seeds used can greatly influence the quality of the oil. High-quality grapeseed oil is typically a clear light yellow-green color, and has a very mild, almost neutral flavor. It's often used for culinary and cosmetic purposes.

3.2 Grapeseed Oil versus Grapeseed Extract

So, you got a hankering to know what's the difference between grapeseed oil and grapeseed extract, right?

Back in the day, I was as clueless as a tumbleweed about grapeseed oil and extract until Paul Harvey spilled the beans on his radio show, "The Rest of The Story" . Even then, I was left scratching my head, wondering what in tarnation it was. With the internet not as easy to wrangle in the early 2000's, I had to mosey over to the library, chat with folks at the nutrition store, and even powwow with my doctors, yet nuggets of info were as scarce as hen's teeth.

Fast forward to today, the internet's become a vast field of knowledge, and I've corralled below what I know as the important info on grapeseed oil and extract.

So, partner, let's ride on...

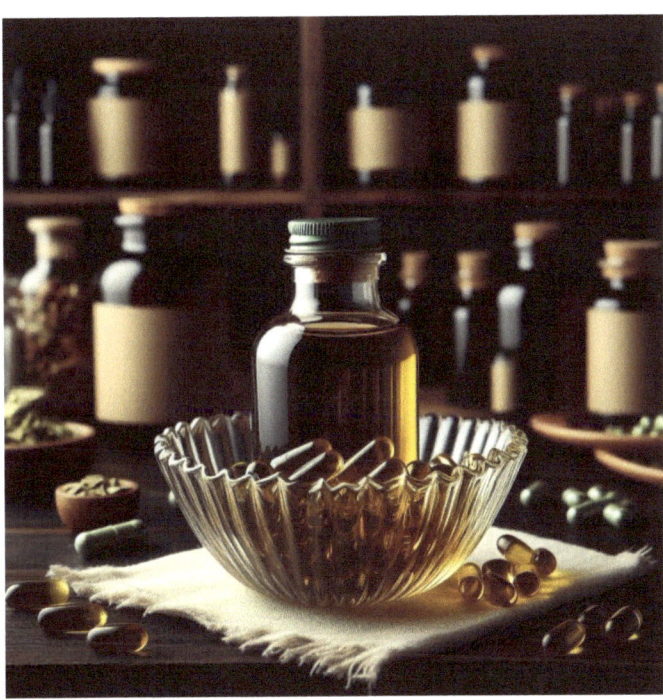

Chrissy Hartmann

3.3 The Grapes

Grapeseed oil and grapeseed extract are derived from the same source but serve different purposes and have distinct characteristics. Here are the key differences and similarities between the two:

Grapeseed Oil

- **Source:** Grapeseed oil is obtained by cold-pressing the seeds of grapes, primarily from wine grapes.

- **Composition:** It is primarily a culinary oil and consists of fatty acids, particularly polyunsaturated fats (such as linoleic acid), monounsaturated fats (like oleic acid), and a small amount of saturated fat. In fact, according to the USDA, one tablespoon of grapeseed oil has about: 14 grams fat (about 10 percent of which is saturated fat, 16 percent monounsaturated and 70 percent polyunsaturated) 120 calories. It also contains 4 milligrams vitamin E (19 percent.

- **Usage:** Grapeseed oil is commonly used in cooking and culinary applications. It has a high smoke point, making it suitable for frying, grilling, sautéing, and baking. It is also used in salad dressings and sauces as a light, neutral-flavored cooking oil.

- **Health Benefits:** Grapeseed oil is often used for its potential health benefits, such as being heart-healthy due to its polyunsaturated fats. It contains vitamin E and other antioxidants. It is also used in some beauty and skincare products for its moisturizing properties.

- **Taste:** Grapeseed oil has a mild, neutral flavor that doesn't overpower the taste of the dishes.

Grapeseed Extract

- **Source:** Like grapeseed oil the extract is derived from various types of grapes, but the most common varieties used for grapeseed oil and grapeseed extract are often Vitis vinifera grapes. These grapes include varieties like Cabernet Sauvignon, Merlot, and Pinot Noir. Grapeseed oil is extracted from the seeds, while grapeseed extract is derived from the crushed seeds and sometimes the skins of these grapes.

Grapeseed Extract
- Composition: It is not an oil but a concentrated supplement or extract. Grapeseed extract is rich in bioactive compounds, including proanthocyanidins, flavonoids, and resveratrol, which are antioxidants and phytochemicals.

- Usage: Grapeseed extract is not used as a cooking or culinary ingredient. It is typically available in the form of dietary supplements or capsules.

- Health Benefits: Grapeseed extract is often taken as a dietary supplement for its potential health benefits in a concentrated form, such as antioxidant properties that may help protect cells from damage caused by free radicals. Remember, though, grapeseed oil does have antioxidants in it to, just not the concentrated amount like the extract.

Both however are associated with various health claims, including improved heart health and potential anti-inflammatory effects.

- Taste: Grapeseed extract is not consumed for its flavor as it has no real flavor due to its properties being encapsulated in a concentrated-pill form.

Chrissy Hartmann

3.4 Grapeseed Production

The decision to use grapes for grapeseed oil or extract often depends on the intended end product and the extraction process. Grapeseed oil is primarily obtained through cold pressing the seeds of wine grapes, with Vitis vinifera varieties being favored for their larger seeds and higher oil content. The choice between oil and extract production is typically made by companies or individuals involved in grape processing, depending on market demand, and intended applications.

As for the main producers of grapeseed oil, countries with significant wine industries often contribute to grapeseed oil and extract production. Major producers include Spain, Italy, France, and the United States of America. These countries benefit from ample grape cultivation and a well-established wine industry who provide a substantial source of grape seeds for extraction.

It's important to note that grapeseed extract, often used as a dietary supplement for its potential health benefits, involves a different extraction process that may include the use of solvents or other methods to concentrate bioactive compounds. The decision to produce grapeseed extract is usually driven by the demand for supplements and health-related products.

3.5 Reasons for Choosing Grapeseed Oil

The extraction method for grapeseed extract typically involves the use of solvents to concentrate beneficial compounds such as proanthocyanidins, polyphenols, and antioxidants. While grapeseed extract is considered safe for consumption when produced according to established quality standards, some people may prefer grapeseed oil for a few reasons:

1. Purity and Simplicity.
Grapeseed oil is often extracted through a simpler cold-pressing method, which may be viewed as a more natural and straightforward process compared to the use of solvents in grapeseed extract production.

2. Less Processing.
Cold pressing retains more of the natural properties of the seeds without the need for additional chemical processes. This can be appealing to those who prefer minimally processed products.

3. Versatility.
Grapeseed oil is widely used in culinary applications and skincare due to its neutral flavor and light texture. It offers a versatile option for cooking and as a base in various beauty products.

While both grapeseed oil and grapeseed extract have their merits, the choice often depends on individual preferences, specific applications, and the desired benefits. It's essential for you cowboys to be aware of the extraction methods used and choose products from reputable sources to ensure safety and quality.

No matter which you choose, both are very healthy.

Chrissy Hartmann

3.6 Grapeseed Antioxidants

And speaking of health, antioxidants play a substantial role in keeping cowboys healthy.
So, what are these antioxidants and their benefits?

Antioxidants are compounds that help neutralize or counteract the damaging effects of free radicals in the body. Free radicals are unstable molecules produced through normal bodily processes and environmental factors like pollution or UV radiation. These molecules can cause oxidative stress, leading to cell damage and potentially contributing to various health issues.

Antioxidant health benefits include:

1. Cell Protection.
Antioxidants neutralize free radicals, protecting cells from damage and reducing the risk of chronic diseases.

2. Heart Health.
They may contribute to cardiovascular health by reducing oxidative stress on blood vessels and lowering inflammation.

3. Cancer Prevention.
Some antioxidants may help prevent or slow the growth of certain cancers by inhibiting oxidative damage to DNA.

4. Anti-Inflammatory Effects.
Antioxidants can have anti-inflammatory properties, helping to manage inflammation in the body.

5. Skin Health.
They play a role in maintaining skin health by protecting against oxidative damage and supporting collagen production.

6. Eye Health.
Certain antioxidants, like lutein and zeaxanthin, are beneficial for eye health and may reduce the risk of age-related macular degeneration.

Common antioxidants include vitamins C and E, beta-carotene, selenium, and various phytochemicals found in fruits, vegetables, nuts, and whole grains. When including a variety of antioxidant-rich foods in your diet, it contributes to overall health and well-being.

Both grapeseed oil and grapeseed extract contain a range of antioxidants, primarily polyphenols and flavonoids.
Here are some of the antioxidants found in both:

1. Proanthocyanidins.
These are a group of flavonoids known for their potent antioxidant properties. Proanthocyanidins are abundant in grapeseed oil and extract.

2. Resveratrol.
This antioxidant has gained attention for its potential health benefits, particularly in to heart health. It's found in the seeds, skin, and stems of grapes.

3. Quercetin.
A flavonoid with antioxidant and anti-inflammatory properties, quercetin is present in both grapeseed oil and extract.

4. Epicatechin.
Another flavonoid, which contributes to the antioxidant profile of grape seeds.

5. Anthocyanins.
While more commonly found in the skin of red and purple grapes, anthocyanins are also present in grapeseed extract.

6. Catechins.
Catechins are a type of flavonoid with antioxidant potential. They are found in both grapeseed oil and extract.

The antioxidants listed above are believed to have various health benefits, including protecting cells from oxidative damage, reducing inflammation, and supporting heart health. It's important to note that the specific composition and concentration of antioxidants can vary depending on the grape variety and the processing methods used to produce grapeseed oil and extract.

Chrissy Hartmann

3.7 Grape Varieties

When it comes to wrangling grapeseed oil and extract, it's the Vitis vinifera varieties that often take the blue ribbon. Let me break it down for ya:

1. Chardonnay:
 - Grown: France, California, Australia
 - Grape Type: White
 - Used For: White wine and grapeseed oil. Known for its neutral taste, Chardonnay seeds are often pressed to extract grapeseed oil, adding a touch of gold to your culinary adventures.

2. Cabernet Sauvignon:
 - Grown: California, Bordeaux, Chile
 - Grape Type: Red
 - Used For: Red wine

3. Sauvignon Blanc:
 - Grown: New Zealand, France, California
 - Grape Type: White
 - Used For: White wine and grapeseed oil. These white grape seeds contribute to the production of a light and versatile touch to your cooking.

4. Merlot:
 - Grown: Bordeaux, California, Italy
 - Grape Type: Red
 - Used For: Red wine and grapeseed extract. These seeds are often employed in packing a punch of potential health benefits.

5. Riesling:
 - Grown: Germany, Alsace, Washington
 - Grape Type: White
 - Used For: White wine and grapeseed extract. These seeds offer a concentrated dose of those good-for-you compounds.

6. Syrah/Shiraz:
 - Grown: Rhône Valley, Australia, California
 - Grape Type: Red
 - Used For: Red wine, grapeseed oil, and grapeseed extract. Versatile and hearty grapes that the seeds qualify for either the oil or the extract.

7. Pinot Grigio/Pinot Gris:
 - Grown: Italy, Oregon, Germany
 - Grape Type: White
 - Used For: White wine

8. Zinfandel:
 - Grown: California, Croatia, Italy
 - Grape Type: Red
 - Used For: Red wine

So, there you have it. Whether you're looking for a cooking companion with grapeseed oil or eyeing the potential health perks in grapeseed extract, these grapes from the Vitis vinifera posse are your go-to.

But hold onto your hat because there's a little more with regards to its nutritional breakdown.

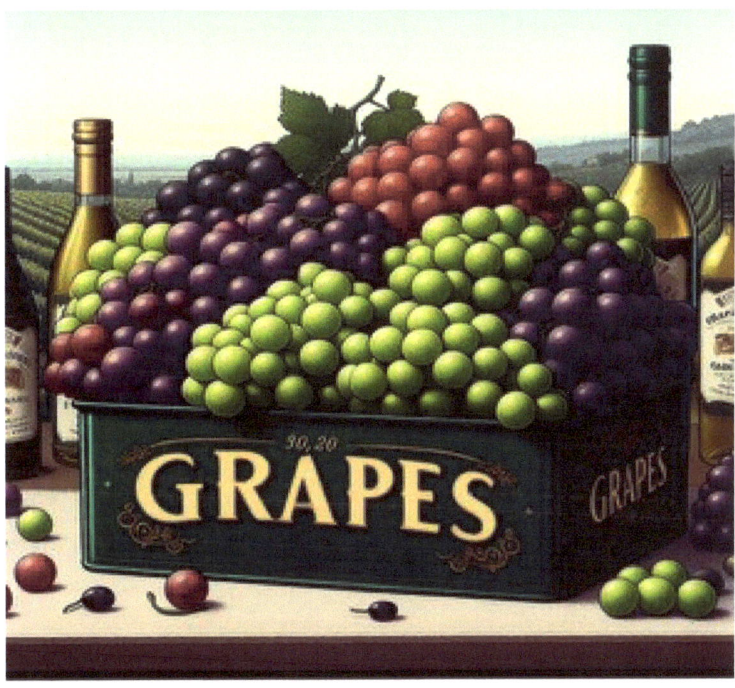

Chrissy Hartmann

3.8 Grapeseed Oil Nutritional Value

Serving Size: 1 tablespoon
Servings: 1
Calories: 120

% Daily value based on a 2000 calorie diet
Total Fat 13.6 grams
Saturated Fat 1.3 grams	10%
Trans Fat 0 grams	0%
Polyunsaturated Fat 9.5 grams	70%
Monounsaturated Fat 2.2 g	16%
Cholesterol 0 mg	0%
Sodium 0 mg	0%
Carbohydrates 120 g	0%
Dietary Fiber 0 g	0%
Total Sugars 0 g	0%
Protein 0 g	0%

3.9 Daily Recommended Allowances

Well, partner, these here values are just rough guidelines, kinda like trail markers. They can shift a bit depending on your personal health, how active you are, and any dietary needs ya might have. Best bet is to mosey on over to a doc or nutritionist for some custom-tailored advice that'll suit you just right.

Recommended Daily Allowance for a 2000 calorie diet.

1. Total Fat RDA: 78 grams. Percentage of total calories: 35% of total daily calories should come from fat.

2. Saturated Fat RDA: Less than 20 grams. Percentage of total calories: Should be less than 10% of total daily calories.

3. Cholesterol RDA: Less than 300 mg per day

4. Sodium RDA: Less than 2,300 mg per day. Note: For those with high blood pressure or heart disease, 1,500 mg is often recommended.

5. Total Carbohydrates RDA: 275 grams: Percentage of total calories: 45-65% of daily calories should come from carbohydrates.

6. Dietary Fiber: RDA: 28 grams

7. Total Sugars: RDA: There is no specific daily value for total sugars. However, added sugars should be limited to: Less than 50 grams (or about 10% of daily calories) according to the FDA.

8. Protein RDA: 50 grams - Percentage of total calories: 10-35% of total daily calories should come from protein.

**Now, don't forget, these numbers are just general recommendations, kinda like a blueprint. Folks' needs can change depending on things like age, gender, and health conditions. So, it isn't one-size-fits-all!

Now, if you want healthy eats, saddle up and head for the kitchen and try your hand at some recipes made with the liquid gold of the grape – grapeseed oil. Trust me, your taste buds will thank you for the adventure. Happy cooking!

Chrissy Hartmann

3.10 Grapeseed Oil — Safe for the Trail if Ridden Right

Well, let me tell ya, over the years, we've heard all kinds of tall tales about what's good for eating and what's not. Coffee? They said it'd keep your heart thumping till it stops for good. Butter? Bad for the blood, they said. And don't get me started on red meat, taters, and dark chocolate—yup, they were supposed to be the devil's own in disguise. And now, they've got their sights set on seed oils, like my old friend, grapeseed oil. But like any chuckwagon cook worth his salt, I've done my research, and let me tell ya, this isn't the boogeyman that they're making it out to be.

Now, I reckon moderation's the name of the game. Sure, seed oils got omega-6 fats, which can cause a stir if you go slathering them on everything in sight. Too much omega-6 can tip the scales toward inflammation. But when you balance it out with omega-3 oils like flaxseed or a good old glug of olive oil, you're sitting pretty. Matter of fact, I even toss a teaspoon of flaxseed into my coffee each morning—keeps things regular and balances that fatty acid ratio like a well-tuned horse. Harvard's nutrition folks back this up, saying it's all about getting the right kinds of fat in a balanced way ([Harvard T.H. Chan School of Public Health](https://www.hsph.harvard.edu/nutritionsource/what-should-you-eat/fats-and-cholesterol/types-of-fat/)).

Grapeseed oil got some other good qualities, too—antioxidants like vitamin E that's kept this old cowboy's heart ticking strong after a scare 10+ years ago, and I'll even credit it for mending my neuropathy something fierce. It's got a high smoke point too, which is mighty handy when you're frying or searing and need something that won't go up in smoke. For folks curious about inflammation, I'd point them to AllRecipes](https://www.allrecipes.com/article/best-and-worst-oils-for-anti-inflammatory-diet and Healthlinehttps://www.healthline.com/nutrition/10-healthy-cooking-oils), which explain how the type of fat matters more than some folks might think.

So long as you don't go hog-wild with it, grapeseed oil's a fair choice in my book. Pair it with whole foods, a balanced diet, and a good dose of common sense, and you'll do just fine. And if you're hankering for more info regarding the benefits of grapeseed oil and how to cook with it, check out the following resources and articles:

1. "Is Grapeseed Oil a Healthy Cooking Oil? Find Out" by Dr. Josh Axe
Summary: This article provides a balanced look at the pros and cons of grapeseed oil, particularly for its use in moderate-heat cooking like stir-fries, sautéing, and baking. Dr. Axe discusses its light flavor, versatility, and benefits when cold-pressed, which preserves its nutrient profile.
URL: [draxe.com] (https://draxe.com/nutrition/grapeseed-oil/)

2. "16 Amazing Benefits of Grapeseed Oil and How to Use It" by Natural Remedy Ideas
Summary: This piece highlights various health benefits of grapeseed oil, including its antioxidant properties, vitamin E content, and immune-supporting capabilities. It also provides tips for using it in recipes, making it ideal for salad dressings, marinades, and light cooking methods.
URL: [naturalremedyideas.com](https://naturalremedyideas.com/benefits-of-grapeseed-oil/)

3. "What Is Grapeseed Oil Good For?" by Healthline
Summary: This article gives an overview of grapeseed oil's health benefits, its fatty acid profile, and why it's best suited for low to medium heat cooking. Healthline also notes its role as an alternative to oils with a stronger taste, allowing other flavors in a dish to shine.
URL: [healthline.com](https://www.healthline.com/nutrition/grapeseed-oil)

4. "What Happens to Your Body When You Eat Grapeseed Oil Regularly" by EatingWell Editors
Summary: This article explores the potential benefits of grapeseed oil, such as promoting cardiovascular health, improving skin, and offering anti-inflammatory effects. It discusses grapeseed oil's omega-6 content, which, when balanced with omega-3s, can be heart-healthy.
URL: [EatingWell](https://www.eatingwell.com/article/8057800/what-happens-to-your-body-when-you-eat-grapeseed-oil-regularly/)

5. "Grape Seed Oil Benefits, Uses, and Side Effects: An In-Depth Guide" by Natural Living Editors
Summary: This article covers grapeseed oil's rich polyphenol content and its benefits for heart health, as well as its usefulness in high-heat cooking. Additionally, it highlights grapeseed oil's anti-inflammatory and antioxidant properties, which support skin health and overall wellness.
URL: [Natural Living Online](https://naturallivingonline.com/grape-seed-oil-benefits-uses-and-side-effects-an-in-depth-guide)

6. "4 Healthy Oils Beyond Olive Oil to Eat Every Week" by Lauren Harris-Pincus, MS, RDN
Summary: This piece explains the benefits of various oils, including grapeseed oil, for their healthy fat profiles and high smoke points, making them suitable for diverse cooking methods. It also mentions that grapeseed oil's vitamin E content can be beneficial when consumed in moderation.
URL: [Nutrition Starring YOU](https://nutritionstarringyou.com/4-healthy-oils-beyond-olive-oil-to-eat-every-week/)

7. "There's No Reason to Avoid Seed Oils and Plenty of Reasons to Eat Them," by Laura Williamson, The American Heart Association

Chrissy Hartmann

Summary: The American Heart Association addresses the misinformation surrounding seed oils and supports the idea that they are a healthy choice, particularly for heart health, based on current scientific evidence.

URL: (Heart.org) (https://www.heart.org/en/news/2024/08/20/theres-no-reason-to-avoid-seed-oils-and-plenty-of-reasons-to-eat-them)

Well now, partner, if you've made it this far, you've heard this here old Chuckwagon cook ramble on about grapeseed oil and all its benefits. But I'm not here to sugarcoat things, I'm just telling you like it is from a good old cowboy's perspective. You see, there's always something out there to stir the pot, especially on social media where folks get all hot under the collar about this or that. But, when you look at the facts, you find that grapeseed oil isn't the enemy folks want to make it out to be. It's got antioxidants, helps the heart and in my personal opinion heals the neuropathy , at least it did for me. And it's been part of my kitchen for years. And my ticker is still kicking as I twostep across the chuckwagon. No heart attacks or troubles since that one back in 2013.

Sure, you gotta be smart about what you're cooking and balance things out with good old whole foods, and some flaxseed never hurt no one either. In my world, moderation and variety keep the body running smooth like a well-oiled chuckwagon. So, don't let all that negativity get under your skin. We're all just here to cook up the best for our grub-hungry cowboys—feed 'em hearty, feed them right. No need to fear a little grapeseed oil in your pan, folks. Just keep it balanced, and you should be just fine.

Happy cooking you all. And remember—this here's just the grumpy cowboy cook's take. If you want the science behind it, go ahead and take a gander at the articles above like this one here on Heart.org, which has more on seed oils and heart health https://www.heart.org/en/news/2024/08/20/theres-no-reason-to-avoid-seed-oils-and-plenty-of-reasons-to-eat-them.

Still feeling a little unsure? Well, don't just take my word for it. If you're worried about how seed oils might fit into your diet or health plan, it's always a clever idea to have a chat with your family doctor, nutritionist, or dietitian. Those folks are there to steer you right and answer any of them questions you might have. Stay healthy, stay hungry, and remember: a full belly makes a happy cowboy.

Chapter 4 Sunrise Delights

Around these parts, breakfast is the most important meal of the day. It's what fuels us for a day of hard work whether it's riding the pastures fixing fences, or rounding up the herd to brand the cattle.

So throw in some grapeseed oil in your mornings to enhance the raw flavors of your breakfast and lasso in those health benefits.

Grapeseed oil is known here in these parts for its light, neutral taste and numerous health benefits, making it the jack of all oils as a selection for various breakfast recipes.

So, why not start your day out with an extra jingle to your spurs?

Adding grapeseed oil into your breakfast recipes not only gives that extra giddy up to its taste but also boosts the nutritional value of your morning meal.

Grab a cup of coffee and enjoy your delicious and nutritious breakfast while you watch the sunrise bloom!

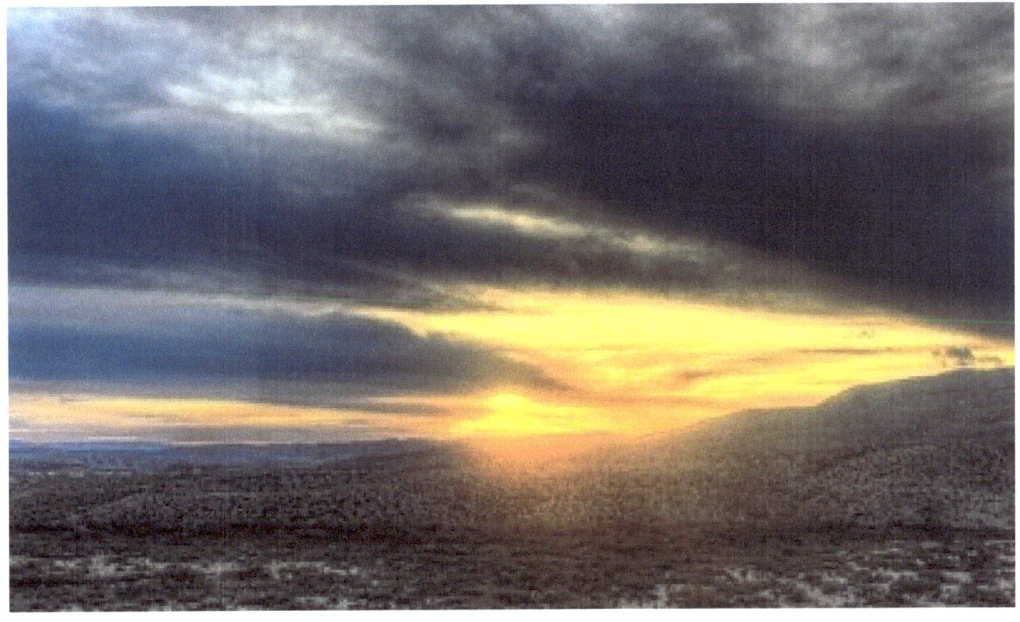

Chrissy Hartmann

4.1 Blueberry Flapjacks

Serving Size: 2
Servings: 10
Approximate Calories: 247

Ingredients:
- 2 cups all-purpose flour
- 2 tablespoons sugar
- 2 teaspoons baking powder
- 1 teaspoon baking soda
- Optional: 1/2 teaspoon salt
- 2 eggs
- 2 cups buttermilk
- 4 tablespoons grapeseed oil
- 2 cups fresh blueberries

Instructions:
1. In a mixing bowl, Sift the flour so it resembles desert sand with the sugar, baking powder, baking soda, and salt.
2. In another bowl, beat the eggs, then add buttermilk and grapeseed oil. Mix until well combined.
3. Pour the wet ingredients into the dry ingredients and stir until just combined.
4. Gently fold in the fresh blueberries like a graceful dance partner.
5. Heat a heavy skillet over medium-high heat and lightly grease with grapeseed oil.
6. Pour 1/4 cup portions of the flapjack batter onto the griddle.
7. Cook until bubbles form on the surface, then Flip flapjacks with a flick of the wrist and cook until golden brown.
8. Serve with maple syrup and extra blueberries.

Nutrition Value:
% Daily Value based on a 2000 calorie diet
Total Fat 8.9 g	11%
Saturated Fat 1.4 g	7%
Cholesterol 43 mg	14%
Sodium 388 mg	17%
Carbohydrates 35.7 g	13%
Dietary Fiber 1.8 g	6%
Total Sugars 9.7 g	
Protein 6.9 g	

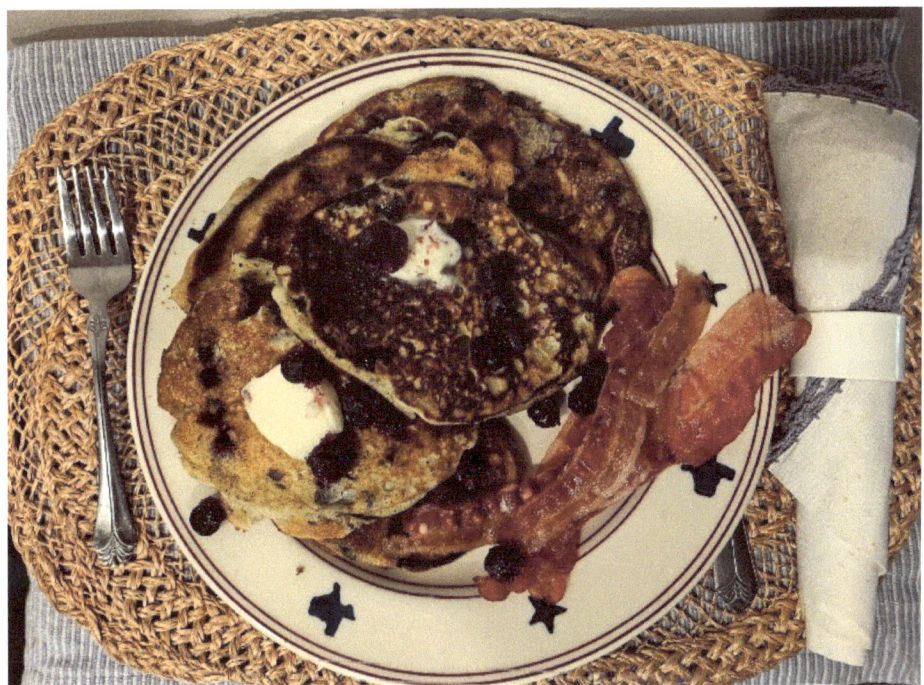

Grumbles from the Chuckwagon:
Let's just say that the cowboys around here love waking up to the fiery sunrises, but better yet, when they sidle up to a plate of these blueberry flapjacks, they're nothing but thankful. And we here in the chuckwagon appreciate the high heat point of grapeseed oil, because sometimes cooking over a flame might get hotter than planned.

Chrissy Hartmann

4.2 Healthy Morning Smoothie

Serving Size: 12 oz
Servings: 2
Approximate Calories: 323

Ingredients:
- 1 cup mixed berries (strawberries, blueberries, raspberries)
- 1 ripe banana
- 1/2 cup Greek yogurt
- 1 tablespoon honey
- 1 tablespoon grapeseed oil
- 1/2 cup almond or oat milk
- Ice cubes

Instructions:
1. Add the mixed berries, banana, Greek yogurt, honey, and grapeseed oil to a blender.
2. Pour in almond or oat milk and add ice cubes.
3. Blend until smooth and creamy.
4. Pour into a glass and enjoy your nutrient-packed smoothie.

Nutritional Value:
% Daily Value based on a 2000 calorie diet

Total Fat 21.5 g	28%
Saturated Fat 13.4 g	67%
Cholesterol 0 mg	0%
Sodium 10 mg	0%
Carbohydrates 34 g	12%
Dietary Fiber 5.4 g	19%
Total Sugars 22.8 g	
Protein 2.5 g	

Grumbles from the Chuckwagon:
Sipping on this fruit smoothie while the sun comes up feels like wrangling a herd of flavors with the taste of sunshine Turning this breakfast into a roundup of freshness that hits the trail just right. And speaking of the trail, I've got more giddy up with this and some granola that my own pony looks at me in wide-eyed bewilderment.

4.3 Western Sunrise Slices

Serving Size: 2 slices
Servings: 2
Approximate Calories: 231

Ingredients:
- 4 slices of hardy bread
- 2 eggs
- 1/2 cup oat milk
- 1 teaspoon pure vanilla extract
- 1 tablespoon grapeseed oil
- Ground cinnamon (to taste)
- Maple syrup for serving

Instructions:
1. In bowl, whisk together eggs, milk, vanilla, and a pinch of ground cinnamon.
2. Heat skillet over medium heat, add grapeseed oil.
3. Dip each slice of hardy bread into the egg mixture, allowing it to soak for a moment.
4. Place the hardy bread in the skillet and cook until golden brown on both sides.
5. Serve with a drizzle of maple syrup.

Nutritional Value:
% Daily Value based on a 2000 calorie diet

Total Fat 12.4 g	16%
Saturated Fat 2.3 g	12%
Cholesterol 188 mg	63%
Sodium 258 mg	11%
Carbohydrates 16 g	6%
Dietary Fiber 0.6 g	2%
Total Sugars 7.5 g	
Protein 11.7 g	

Grumbles from the Chuckwagon:
Devouring these here western sunrise slices is like roping in a taste of heaven at daybreak. The sweet swirl of cinnamon and the golden-brown perfection of each hardy slice make a cowboy's morning as satisfying as a successful cattle drive under the big blue sky.

Chrissy Hartmann

4.4 Saddle Hearty Oatmeal

Serving Size: 1 bowl
Servings: 2
Approximate Calories: 431

Ingredients:
- 2 cups rolled oats
- 4 cups water
- Optional: 1/4 teaspoon salt
- 2 tablespoons grapeseed oil
- 2 Tablespoons ground Flaxseed
- Fresh berries and honey for topping

Instructions:
1. In a saucepan, bring water to a boil, then add oats, ground flaxseed, and salt.
2. Reduce heat and simmer, stirring occasionally, until oats are creamy.
3. Stir in grapeseed oil and cook for another minute.
4. Serve hot, topped with fresh berries and a drizzle of honey.

Nutritional Value:
% Daily Value based on a 2000 calorie diet

Total Fat 13.3 g	17%
Saturated Fat 1.7 g	9%
Cholesterol 0 mg	0%
Sodium 13 mg	1%
Carbohydrates 64.3 g	23%
Dietary Fiber 9.8 g	35%
Total Sugars 7.9 g	
Protein 11.6 g	

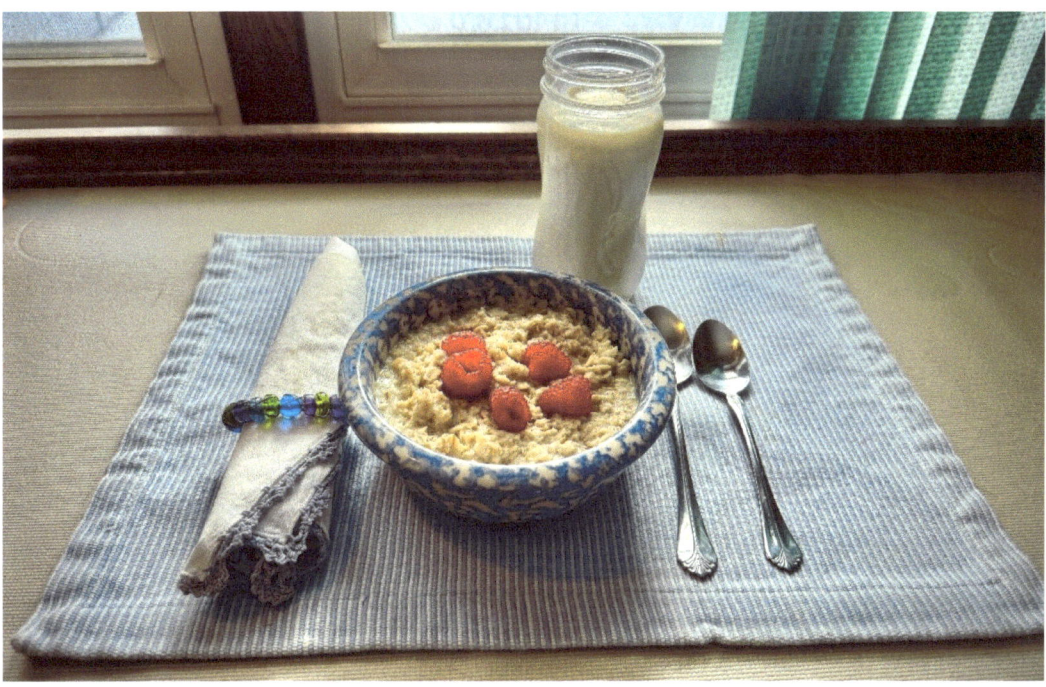

Grumbles from the Chuckwagon:
Making this oatmeal is as straightforward as riding a well-broke horse. Just boil water, toss in oats, grapeseed oil, and that there ground flaxseed, and let simmer like a prairie sunset and voila! Easy as roping a calf on a lazy afternoon. And don't forget about the hardiness of it. Remember this here in your belly will enable you to sit tall in your saddle with the best of them.

Chrissy Hartmann

4.5 Western Banana-Cran Bites

Serving Size: 1
Servings: 12
Approximate Calories: 153

Ingredients:
- 3 ripe bananas, mashed
- 1/3 cup grapeseed oil
- 1/2 cup brown sugar
- 1 egg
- 1 teaspoon vanilla extract
- 1 1/2 cups all-purpose flour
- 1/2 teaspoon baking soda
- 1 1/2 teaspoons baking powder
- 1 cup fresh cranberries

Instructions:
1. Preheat oven to 350°F. Grease muffin tin.
2. In bowl, combine mashed bananas, grapeseed oil, sugar, egg, and vanilla extract.
3. In another bowl, Sift the flour to resemble desert sand with baking soda, and baking powder. Then add to banana mixture.
4. Then fold in cranberries like a graceful dance partner.
5. Spoon batter into muffin cups and bake for 18-20 minutes, or until a toothpick comes out clean.

Nutritional Value:
% Daily Value based on a 2000 calorie diet
Total Fat 3.8 g   5%
Saturated Fat 0.6 g   3%
Cholesterol 31 mg   10%
Sodium 1166 mg   51%
Carbohydrates 25.2 g   9%
Dietary Fiber 1.4 g   5%
Total Sugars 7.5 g
Protein 2.5 g

Grumbles from the Chuckwagon:
In a quandary here. My cowboys love chowing down on these flavorful muffins of tangy cranberries and sweet bananas. With one bite, their flavors make you feel like you're sweeping across the open range like puffy clouds. But the boss herd asked me not to make any more. Why? Reckon it's cause too much chowing and not enough herding. He's already had to wrangle a few of them heifers away from those randy bulls by himself. Ahh, got to love the bites of western life.

4.6 Cowboy Granola Crunch

Serving Size: 1 cup
Servings: 5
Approximate Calories: 643

Ingredients:
- 3 cups rolled oats
- 1/4 cup grapeseed oil
- 1/2 cup sliced almonds
- 1/2 cup chopped walnuts
- 1/2 cup honey
- 1 teaspoon vanilla extract
- 1 cup dried fruit (cranberries, apricots, raisins, et cetera)

Instructions:
1. Preheat oven to 325°F.
2. In large bowl, combine oats and chopped nuts.
3. In small saucepan, warm honey, grapeseed oil, and vanilla extract over low heat.
4. Pour honey-oil mixture over the oats and nuts, stir to coat evenly.
5. Spread mixture on baking sheet and bake for 20-25 minutes, stir occasionally until golden.
6. Once cool, mix in dried fruit and store in an airtight container.

Nutritional Value:
% Daily Value based on a 2000 calorie diet

Total Fat 35.8 g	46%
Saturated Fat 3.1 g	15%
Cholesterol 0 mg	0%
Sodium 5 mg	0%
Carbohydrates 71.3 g	26%
Dietary Fiber 10.1 g	36%
Total Sugars 31.6 g	
Protein 15.8 g	

Chrissy Hartmann

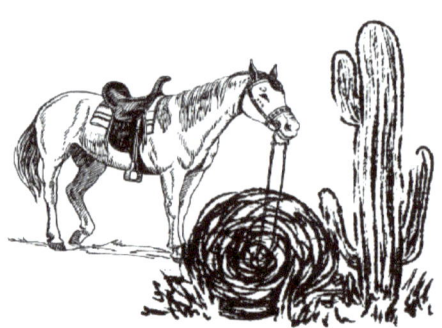

Grumbles from the Chuckwagon:
As the sun spread its golden glow across the horizon, I watched from the chuckwagon as the young cowboys gathered around. They had coffee in one hand an in the other my Cowboy Granola Crunch aiming to lure the attention of the cowgirls attending to the ponies. Little did those young guns know it wasn't their cowboy charm doing the trick, it was my darn good granola. The aroma wafted through the air captivating not the cowgirls, but their ponies who wandered over with curious eyes. There I stood chuckling behind the pots and pans realizing today that it was the granola that stole the show. See in the chuckwagon, it's the flavors that do the talking and this morning they spoke louder than any cowboy's smooth talking. Sorry boys, better luck next time.

4.7 Texas Steak and Egg Fajita

Serving Size: 1 fajita
Servings: 4
Approximate Calories: 329

Ingredients:
- 8 ounces steak, cut into strips
- 4 large eggs
- 1 Tablespoon grapeseed oil
- 4 ounces shredded cheddar cheese
- 1 green pepper, seeded and diced
- 1 teaspoon Chipotle Seasoning
- Salsa and sour cream to garnish

Instructions:
1. Scramble eggs in small bowl.
2. Deseed green pepper and dice. Add to scrambled eggs mixture with chipotle seasoning.
3. In heavy skillet heat up grapeseed oil. Brown steak strips to an internal temperature of 165°F.
4. Add egg mixture to steak and scramble over medium high heat.
5. Spoon steak and egg mixture on to corn tortilla shell and add the shredded cheddar cheese, wrap and fold ends.
6. Plate up with a side of salsa and sour cream.

Nutritional Value:
% Daily Value based on a 2000 calorie daily diet

Total Fat 18 g	23%
Saturated Fat 4.5 g	18%
Cholesterol 138 mg	46%
Sodium 58 mg	3%
Carbohydrates 5.4 g	2%
Dietary Fiber 0 g	0%
Total Sugars 0.2 g	
Protein 22 g	

Grumbles from the Chuckwagon:
When those Texas steak and egg fajitas joined the breakfast repertoire, it stirred up a morning whirlwind. I found myself up with the sun, fixing up that there sizzling steak, melted cheddar, and green peppers to be wrapped in a corn tortilla. Regardless of the challenging day ahead, the mere mention of those fajitas transformed weary eyes into eager early risers. The chuck wagon metamorphosed into a breakfast haven, and before the sun fully ascended, plates were generously heaped with flavors that effortlessly swept away yesterday's hardships warming my ticker.

Chrissy Hartmann

4.8 Feta Fiesta Spinach Eggs

Serving Size: 1 cup
Servings: 2
Approximate Calories: 265

Ingredients:
- 4 large eggs
- 1 tablespoon grapeseed oil
- 1 cup fresh spinach, chopped
- 1/2 cup red bell peppers
- 1/4 cup sliced baby Bella mushrooms
- 1/4 cup crumbled feta cheese
- Salt and pepper to taste

Instructions:
1. In bowl, whisk the eggs until well beaten. Season with a pinch of salt and pepper.
2. Heat non-stick skillet over medium heat and add grapeseed oil.
3. Add the chopped veggies to the skillet and sauté for a minute or until wilted.
4. Pour beaten eggs into skillet and gently stir. Cook until mostly set.
5. Sprinkle crumbled feta cheese over eggs and continue to cook until cheese is melted.
6. Serve hot with whole-grain toast or as filling for a breakfast burrito.
7. Garnish with salsa and sour cream

Nutritional Facts:
% Daily Value based on a 2000 calorie diet

Total Fat 20.9 g	27%
Saturated Fat 6.6 g	33%
Cholesterol 389 mg	130%
Sodium 363 mg	16%
Carbohydrates 4 g	1%
Dietary Fiber 0.7 g	3%
Total Sugars 2.7 g	
Protein 16.3 g	

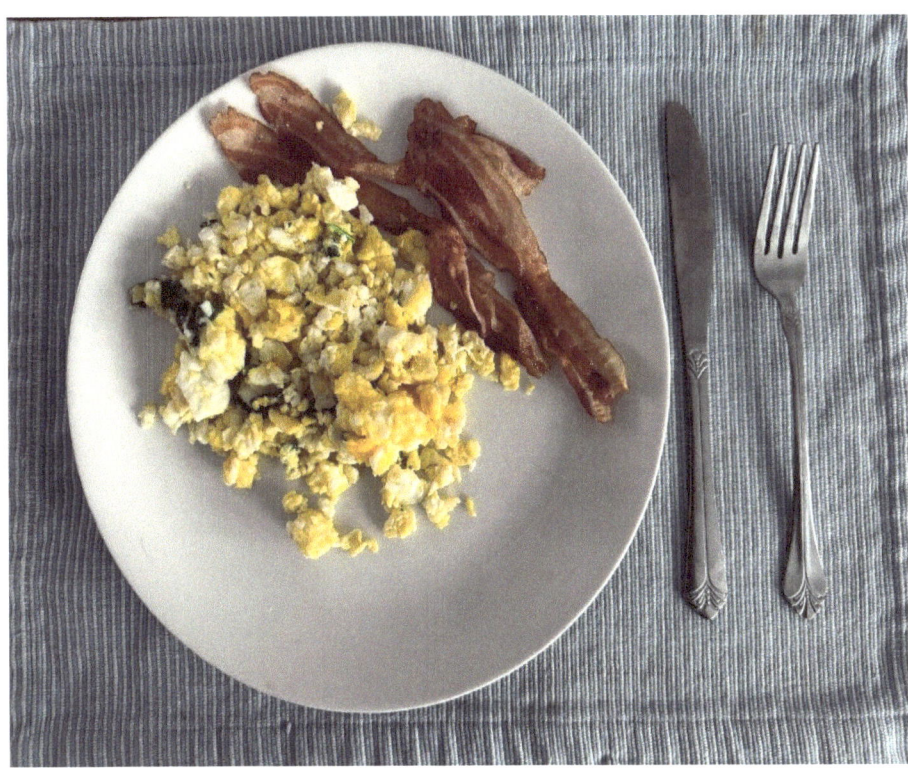

Grumbles from the Chuckwagon:
Not to mince words about these here eggs, but they're fantastic! Even better yet cooked over a campfire with an iron skillet. Just wrap in a tortilla and watch them fly off the plate. Not one of my cowboys have ever turned them down.

Chrissy Hartmann

4.9 Texas Sunshine Muffins

Serving Size: 1 muffin
Servings: 8
Approximate Calories: 244

Ingredients:
- 2 cups all-purpose flour
- 1/2 cup granulated sugar
- 2 teaspoons baking powder
- 1/2 teaspoon baking soda
- Zest and juice of 2 lemons
- 1/4 cup grapeseed oil
- 1 cup Greek yogurt
- 2 large eggs
- 1 teaspoon pure vanilla extract

Instructions:
1. Preheat oven to 375ºF. Grease mini muffin tin.
2. In mixing bowl, sift flour to resemble desert sand and combine sugar, baking powder, and baking soda.
3. In another bowl, whisk together lemon zest, lemon juice, grapeseed oil, Greek yogurt, eggs, and pure vanilla extract.
4. Pour wet ingredients into dry ingredients and stir until just combined.
5. Fill each muffin cup about two-thirds full.
6. Bake for 18-20 minutes or until toothpick comes out clean.
7. Cool and enjoy.

Nutritional Value:
% Daily Value based on a 2000 calorie diet

Total Fat 8.3 g	11%
Saturated Fat 2.3 g	12%
Cholesterol 36 mg	12%
Sodium 98 mg	4%
Carbohydrates 29.1 g	11%
Dietary Fiber 0.7 g	3%
Total Sugars 12.7 g	
Protein 13.6 g	

Grumbles from the Chuckwagon:
This is one fine tasty muffin . A definite favorite while watching the sun rise on the horizon . They're flavored with real lemons that will make your taste buds holler "Yeehaw!" And better yet, add a cup of coffee and you just might ride off with this here chuckwagon cook. But take a number, my saddle is full.

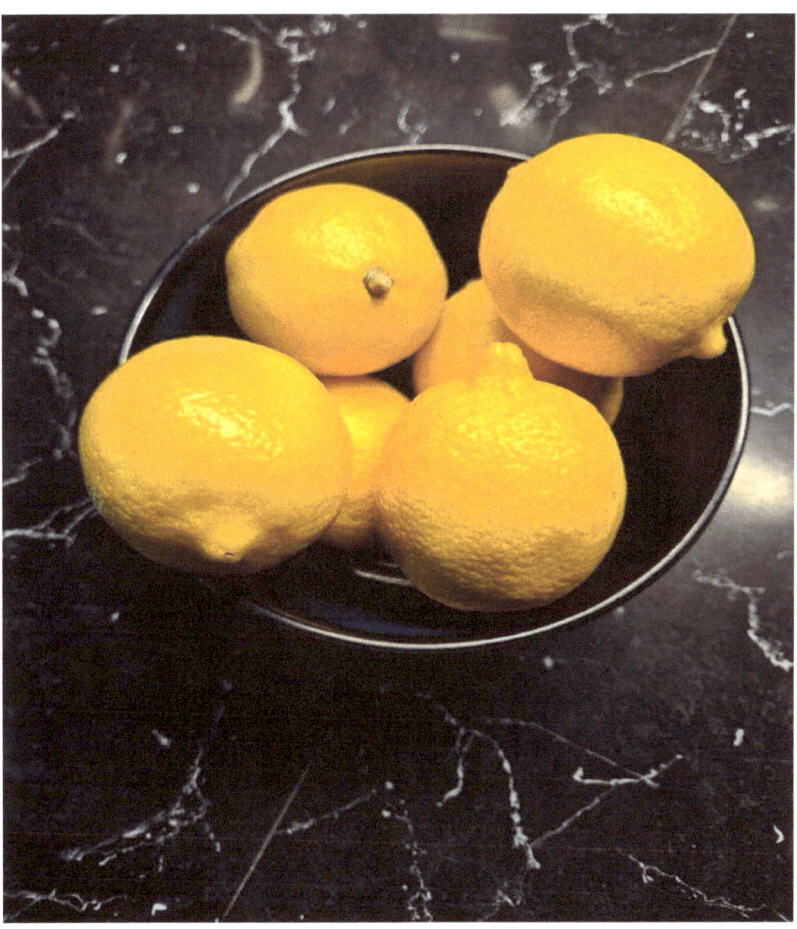

Chrissy Hartmann

4.10 Pumpkin Harvest Berry Bread

Serving Size: 1 Slice
Servings: 12
Approximate Calories: 118

Ingredients:
- Grapeseed Cooking Spray
- 1/2 cup whole wheat pastry flour
- 1/2 cup unbleached all-purpose flour
- 2/3 cup light brown sugar
- 1 teaspoon baking soda
- 1/2 teaspoon salt
- 2 large eggs
- 1 cup canned pumpkin
- 1/4 cup grape seed oil
- 1/2 cup unsweetened applesauce
- 1/4 cup 100% apple juice
- 1/2 teaspoon ground cinnamon
- 1/2 teaspoon ground ginger
- 1/4 ground nutmeg
1/2 cup dried cranberries

Instructions:
1. Preheat oven to 350°F and Lightly coat loaf pan and set aside.
2. In large bowl sift together to resemble desert sand whole wheat pastry flour, all purpose flour, sugar, baking soda, and salt.
3. In medium bowl beat eggs, whisk in pumpkin, grape seed oil, applesauce, apple juice, cinnamon, ginger, and nutmeg.
4. Stir in cranberries.
5. Combine wet and dry ingredients. Mix until all is combined. Do not over stir.
6. Pour into loaf pan and bake for 50 to 60 minutes Letting dough rise like morning sun.
7. Cool on wire rack for 10 minutes.
8. Remove from pan and place on wire rack to continue cooling. Serve warm if desired.

Nutritional Value:
% Daily Value based on a 2000 calorie diet

Total Fat 2.9 g	4%
Saturated Fat 1.2 g	6%
Cholesterol 62 mg	21%
Sodium 3923 mg	171%
Carbohydrates 20.7 g	8%
Dietary Fiber 4.1 g	15%
Total Sugars 7.2 g	
Protein 3.7 g	

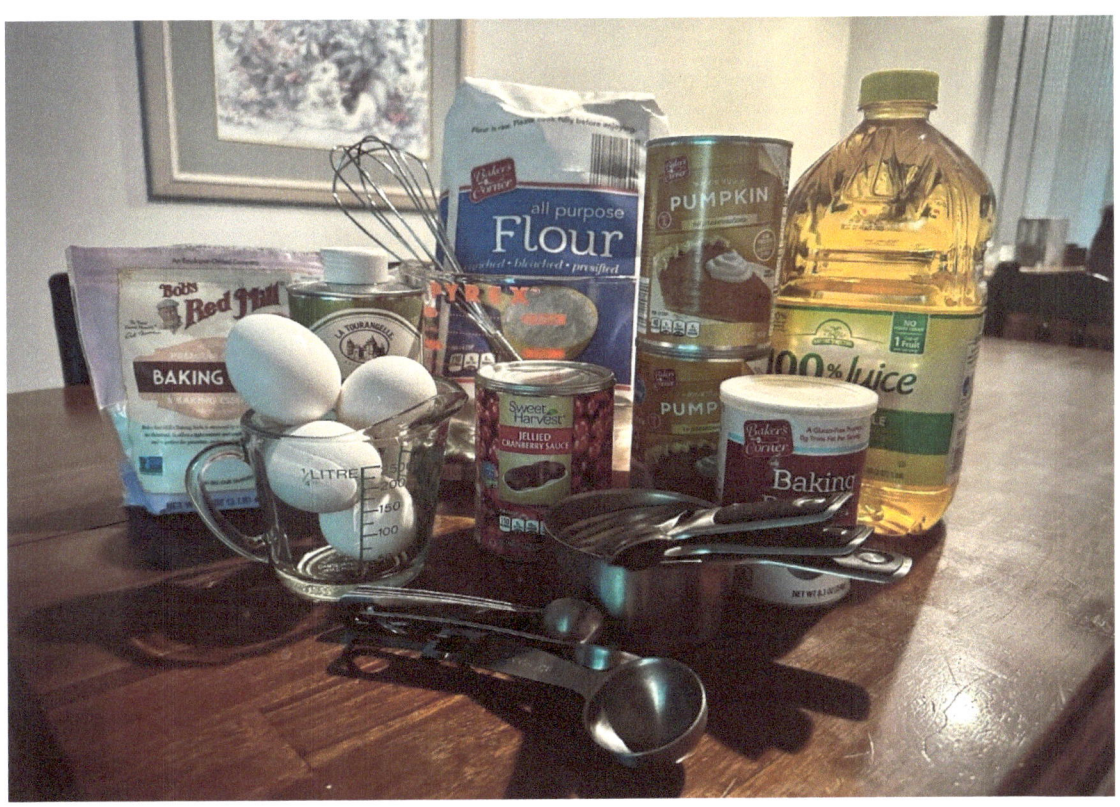

Grumbles from the Chuckwagon:
Ready to cowboy up? Well, you will be after a cup of coffee and this bread. Pumpkin and cranberries aren't just for the fall. Make a loaf and see how many cowboys come knocking on your door. It works! Got mine brewing the coffee and those boys even bought new oven mitts. Yeehaw!

Chrissy Hartmann

The Grub Wrangler's Wisdom:

Chapter 5 Savory Starters

Savory starters set the tone for a great meal, and grapeseed oil can enhance the flavors and nutritional value of your appetizers. Here are some of my delectable recipes along with their respective benefits. But first let me share a story…

Out here in the heart of the West, I have a little secret – my cowboys go wild for my spicy turkey mushrooms. I used to be slick about it, hiding the fact that I was making them, relying on sautéing onions as a decoy scent. But the cowboys caught on, and now the onion trick doesn't fool 'em anymore.

They love those mushrooms more than a gambler loves a winning hand, but a few close calls with fingers in the line of fire made 'em wise up. Now, when that unmistakable fragrance fills the air, the cowboys hold their bellies in check, knowing those mushrooms are hotter than a prairie fire.

It's become a dance of desire and discipline around the chuckwagon. They've learned the hard way that a momentary craving ain't worth the risk of losing a finger or two. So, we share a knowing grin as they resist the temptation, and the tale of my spicy turkey mushrooms becomes a legend in the camp, whispered like the winds across the horizon.

As much as my cowboys love these here savory sides, I hope yours enjoy them as much as I love to make them. Now grab your favorite beverage and sidle up for some good eating!

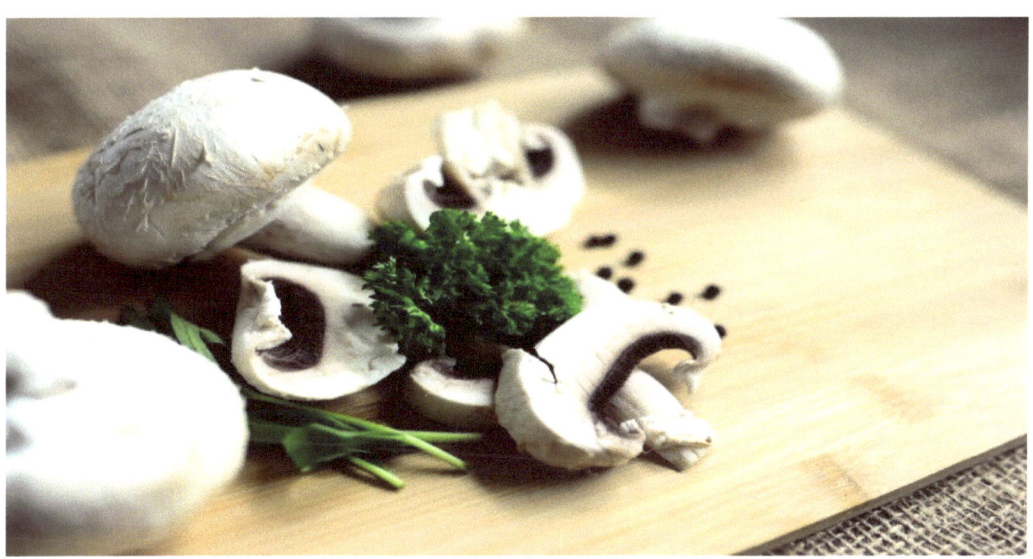

Chrissy Hartmann

5.1 Spicy Hummus with Fresh Veggies

Serving Size: 1 Tablespoon
Servings: 8
Approximate Calories: 109

Ingredients:
- 1 can chickpeas
- 3 tablespoons grapeseed oil
- 2 cloves garlic, minced
- 2 tablespoons ground tahini or substitute with ground sunflower seeds
- Juice of 1 lemon
- 1 teaspoon chili powder
- 1 teaspoon red pepper flakes
- 1 teaspoon cumin
- Salt and black pepper to taste
- Assorted fresh vegetables for dipping

Instructions:
1. Place chickpeas (and juice from can) and minced garlic in pan and cook until softened.
2. In a food processor or blender, combine chickpeas, grapeseed oil, minced garlic, tahini, lemon juice, salt, cumin, chili powder, and red pepper flakes.
3. Blend until smooth and creamy.
4. Serve the hummus with baked pita chips or a variety of fresh vegetables like carrot sticks, cucumber slices, and bell pepper strips.

Nutritional Value:
% Daily Value based on a 2000 calorie diet

Total Fat 3.3 g	4%
Saturated Fat 0.4 g	2%
Cholesterol 0 mg	0%
Sodium 7 mg	0%
Carbohydrates 15.5 g	6%
Dietary Fiber 4.5 g	16%
Total Sugars 2.7 g	
Protein 5.1 g	

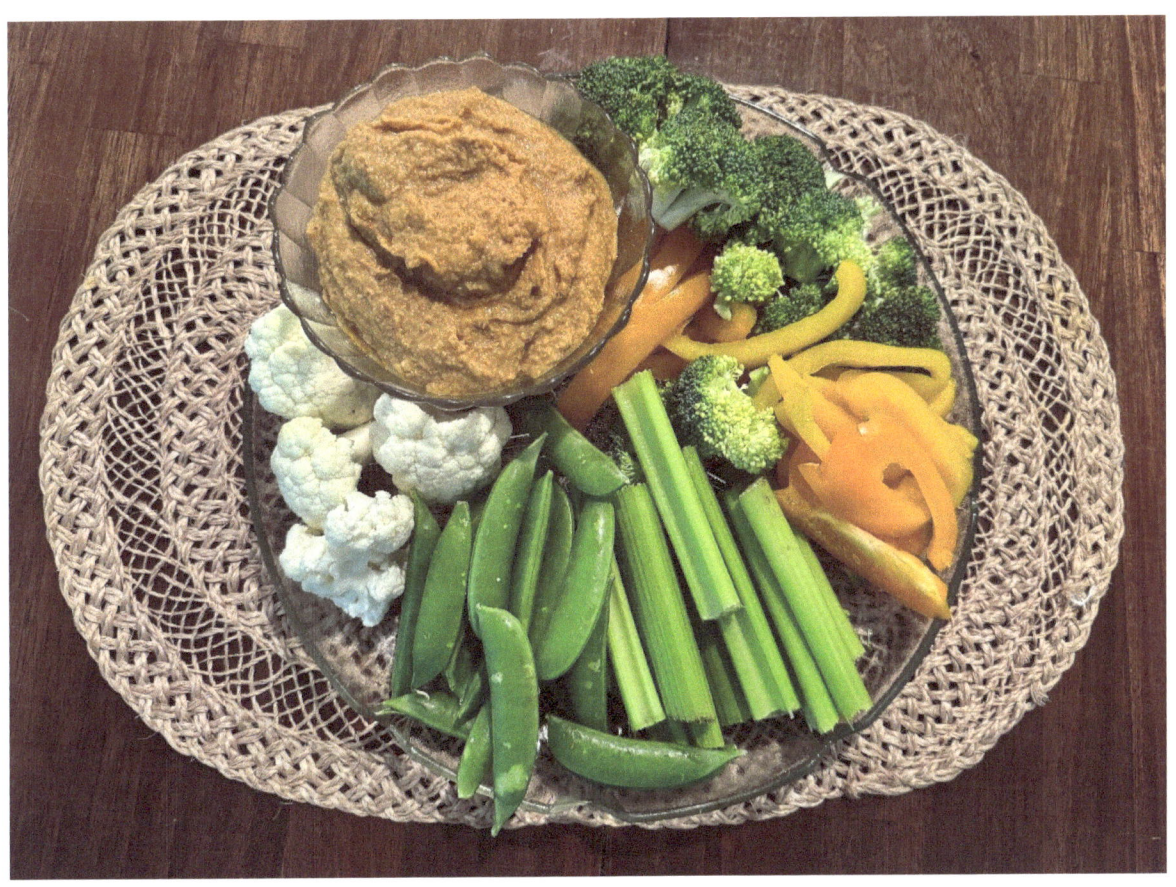

Grumbles from the Chuckwagon:
Boy howdy! here's one of my favorites. It's a quickdraw for your taste buds adding flavor and a fresh crunch -- a tasty pitstop on the trail to a hearty meal. And don't be surprised if you find your cowboys slathering this here dip onto their sandwiches. Quite the topper for turkey and swiss. In fact, two of my cowboys got into a tussle over the last of this here spicy hummus. Needless to say, while they rolled around on the floor wrestling for the container I had more made in the fridge, but hey, it's a hoot to have a show with dinner once in a while.

Chrissy Hartmann

5.2 Butternut Chipotle Turkey Chili

Serving Size: 1 bowl
Servings: 6
Approximate Calories: 722

Ingredients:
- 2 tablespoons grapeseed oil
- 1 pound ground turkey, cooked
- 1 medium red onion, chopped
- 2 red bell peppers, chopped
- 1 small butternut squash, peeled and chopped
- 4 garlic cloves, minced
- 1 tablespoon chili powder
- 1-1/ tablespoons chipotle powder
- 2 cans black beans, rinsed and drained
- 1 small can diced tomatoes
- 2 cups vegetable broth
- corn tortilla chips

Instructions:
1. In a 4- to 6-quart Dutch oven over medium heat, warm the grapeseed oil. Add the onion, bell pepper and butternut squash and cook, stirring occasionally, until onions are translucent.
2. Turn heat to medium-low and add the cooked ground turkey, garlic, chili powder, chipotle powder, smoked paprika, cumin, and cinnamon. Stir constantly until fragrant.
3. Add black beans, canned tomatoes, and veggie broth. Stir occasionally to combine. Cover 1 hour.
4. Add salt to taste
5. Ladle into cups, top with tortilla chips and serve warm.

Nutritional Value:
% daily value based on a 2000 calorie diet
Total Fat 44 g   56%
Saturated Fat 4.7 g   23%
Cholesterol 17 mg   6%
Sodium 340 mg   15%
Carbohydrates 75.2 g   27%
Dietary Fiber 20.9 g   75%
Total Sugars 8 g
Protein 24.1 g

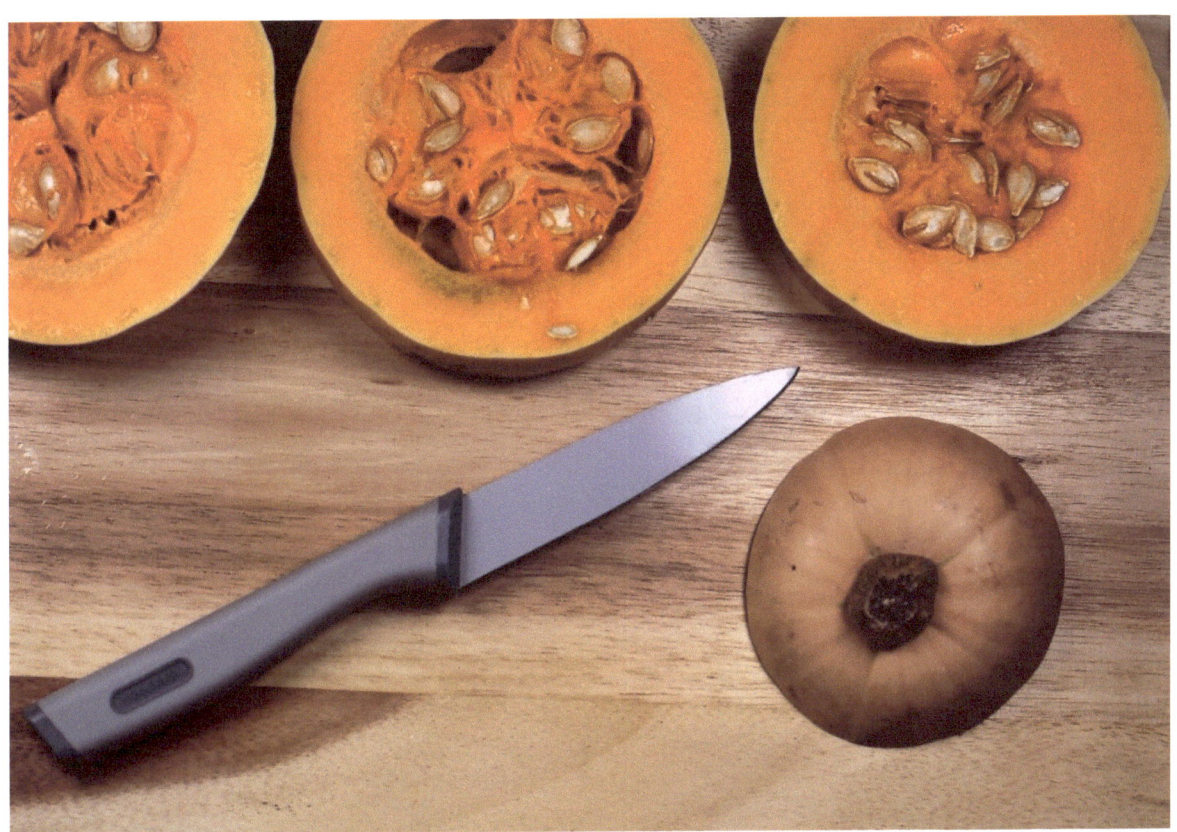

Grumbles from the Chuckwagon:
Long ago some chilies ran wild in this part of the west. Wild and naked. Yep, that's right, meatless. Not taking too kindly to that, this here chuckwagon crew roped us a good one. But the need to break the nakedness came strong. If we wanted our cowboys to chow down on chili, it had to be dressed. So, turkey fit the bill for our healthy appeal. We made both ways, but let me tell ya, when those boys sank their spoons into a bowl of this here Butternut Chipotle Turkey Chili, there spurs began to jingle and their boots started dancing like Saturday night at the saloon. One taste and they were hollering– more turkey in the chili. And let me tell ya, that's the sure-fire secret to keeping those cowpokes happy and fueled up for the day. Now, cowboy up and get cooking!

Chrissy Hartmann

5.3 Robust Spinach Artichoke Dip

Serving Size: 1 Tablespoon
Servings: 8
Approximate Calories: 86

Ingredients:
- 1 cup frozen chopped spinach, thawed and drained
- 1 cup canned artichoke hearts, drained and chopped
- 1/2 cup mayonnaise (See chapter 9 for Homemade Mayo recipe)
- 1/2 cup grated Parmesan cheese
- 1/4 cup grated mozzarella cheese
- 2 cloves garlic, minced
- 1/2 cup shredded cheddar cheese
- 2 tablespoons grapeseed oil

Instructions:
1. Preheat the oven to 350°F.
2. In bowl, combine spinach, artichoke hearts, mayo, Parmesan, mozzarella, and minced garlic.
3. Drizzle grapeseed oil over the mixture and stir to combine.
4. Transfer the mixture to a baking dish and bake for 25-30 minutes until bubbly.
5. Sprinkle the shredded cheddar cheese on top for the last 5 minutes of baking until golden.
6. Serve with toasted pita bread.

Nutritional Value:
% Daily Value based on a 2000 calorie diet

Total Fat 6.8 g	9%
Saturated Fat 1 g	5%
Cholesterol 4 mg	1%
Sodium 132 mg	6%
Carbohydrates 6.1 g	2%
Dietary Fiber 1.2 g	4%
Total Sugars 1.2 g	
Protein 1.2 g	

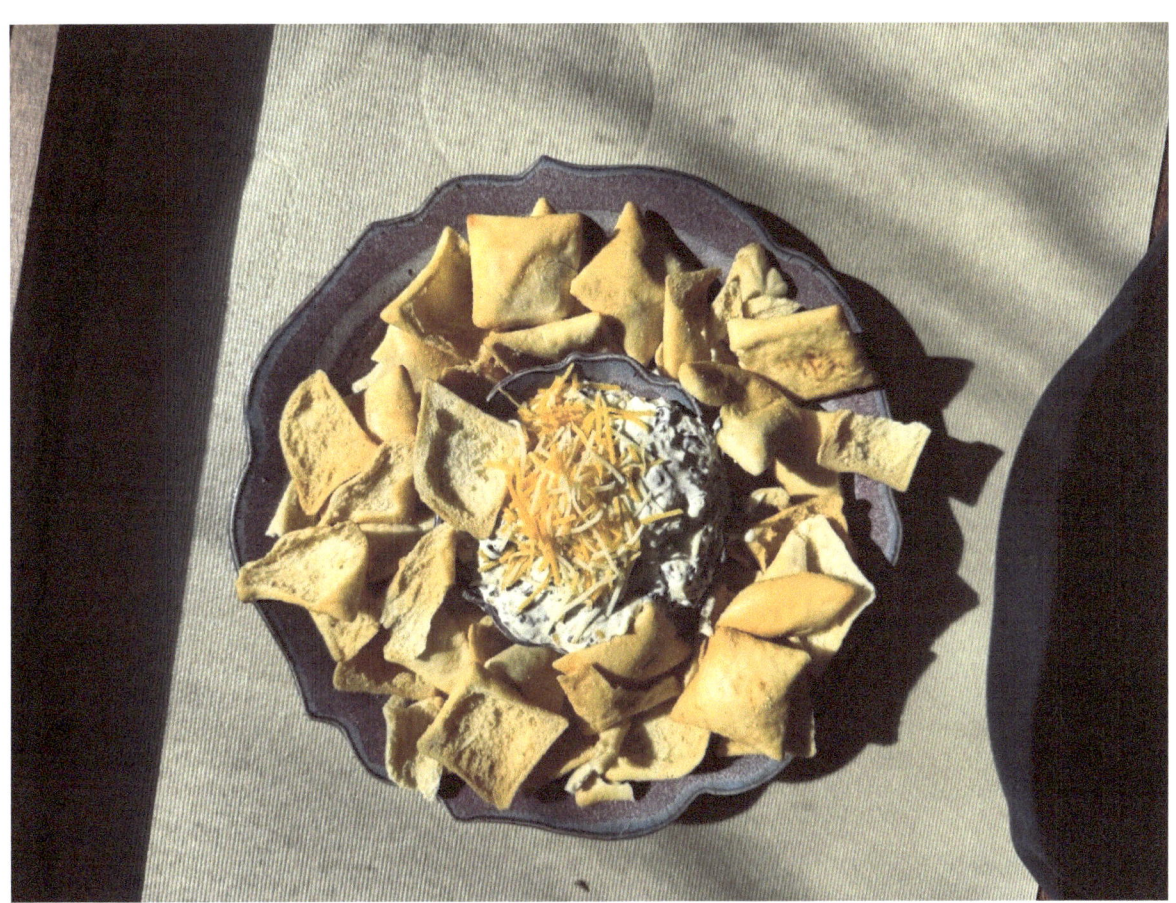

Grumbles from the Chuckwagon:
Nothing like shooting the breeze with your friends and sharing some adult beverages and this here robust dip after a long day out on the range or wrangling a chuckwagon full of dirty pots and pans. This here cheesy crunch will fill you from tip to tail when you don't feel like chowing on anything else. And swirling it in baked pita bread is one two-step the cowboys love to partake in.

Chrissy Hartmann

5.4 Smokey Orange Cauliflower Wings

Serving Size: 1 wing
Servings: 24
Approximate Calories: 142

Ingredients:
- 1 medium head of cauliflower cut into pieces
- 1 pinch of black pepper
- 3 eggs
- 1/2 cup almond flour
- 1 ¼ teaspoon Himalayan salt
- 1/4 teaspoon cayenne pepper
- 3/4 teaspoon garlic powder
- 1 teaspoon smoked paprika
- 2 Tablespoons cornstarch
- 1 spray bottle grapeseed oil
- Orange glaze (see chapter 9)

Instructions:
1. Preheat oven or air fryer to 400°F and line large baking sheet with parchment paper.
2. Add cauliflower florets to large mixing bowl and season with sea salt and black pepper
3. Crack eggs into shallow bowl and whisk until combined. Set aside.
4. Add almond flour, salt, cayenne pepper, garlic powder, paprika, and corn starch and sift together to resemble desert sand. Pour into shallow bowl.
5. Dip cauliflower florets into eggs, coat well, then dip into almond mixture and coat evenly, transfer to parchment-lined baking sheet.
6. Spray evenly with grapeseed oil to crisp coating.
7. Bake for 20 minutes or until golden brown.
8. Transfer cauliflower to large mixing bowl, pour hot orange sauce over top, and gently toss.
9. Serve immediately with celery and blue cheese dressing.

NUTRITIONAL VALUE:
% daily value based on a 2000 calorie diet

Total Fat 7.3 g	9%
Saturated Fat 1 g	5%
Cholesterol 47 mg	16%
Sodium 41 mg	2%
Carbohydrates 16.9 g	6%
Dietary Fiber 4.2 g	15%
Total Sugars 3.1 g	
Protein 4.6 g	

Grumbles from the Chuckwagon:

Before hitting the dance floor for a good old boot scooting boogie, the cowboys eyed the smokey orange cauliflower wings skeptically. This appetizer wasn't their usual fair for a night dancing, but after a day branding cattle, hunger spoke louder than tradition. Reluctantly they dug in. The first bite brought a wave of surprise and as the smokey flavor mingled with the zesty orange glaze, their initial reservation melted away. With a wink and a few nods to me, laughter filled the air and the cauliflower wings disappeared faster than tumbleweeds in the breeze. Turns out a pre-booting bite of the unexpected was just the fuel they needed for a night of two-stepping under the stars. Yeehaw!

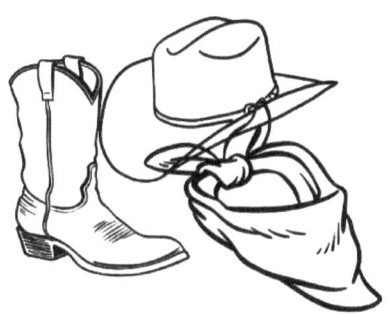

Chrissy Hartmann

5.5 Rustic Chili Potato Wedges

Serving Size: 8 wedges
Servings: 4
Approximate Calories: 319

Ingredients:
- 4 large cleaned russet potatoes, cut into wedges
- 3 tablespoons grapeseed oil
- 2 teaspoons garlic powder
- 2 teaspoon chili powder
- 2 teaspoon onion powder
- Sea salt and black pepper to taste

Instructions:
1. Preheat the oven to 400°F.
2. Cut the potatoes into wedges and soak in warm water for 10 minutes, blot dry.
3. In bowl, toss potato wedges with grapeseed oil, garlic, onion and chili powder, salt, and pepper.
4. Spread the wedges on baking sheet in a single layer. Bake for 30 minutes, turning once, then finish baking for another 30 minutes or until golden and crispy.
5. Serve with salsa, sour cream, and bacon bits.

Nutritional Value:
% Daily Value based on a 2000 calorie diet

Total Fat 7.3 g	9%
Saturated Fat 0.8 g	4%
Cholesterol 0 mg	0%
Sodium 23 mg	1%
Carbohydrates 58.8 g	21%
Dietary Fiber 9.1 g	33%
Total Sugars 4.3 g	
Protein 6.3 g	

Grumbles from the Chuckwagon:
The cowboys huddled near the crackling fire, reminiscing about the glory days of bronco-busting and cattle branding, No one noticed me at first, but when the sweet spicy smell of chili fragranted the air, all the chatter froze. Not even the crickets spoke. I unveiled a piping-hot platter of rustic chili potato wedges. A low whistle accentuated the quiet. The cowboys jumped up. Fingers flew over the platter. They sank their teeth into the crispy wonders and the momentary silence broke with the crunching. I smirked, *who knew these taters could steal the show?*

5.6 Grilled Veggie Bob

Serving Size: 1 veggie-Bob
Servings: 12
Approximate Calories: 184

Ingredients:
- 12 small red potatoes
- 12 cherry tomatoes
- 12 whole baby Bella mushrooms
- 1 green bell pepper sliced
- 1 Vedalia onion sliced
- 1 Zucchinis cubed
- 1/4 cup grapeseed oil
- Papa Fike's Original Seasoning

Instructions:
1. Preheat the grill to 400°F.
2. Cut vegetables into bite-sized pieces.
3. Drizzle grapeseed oil over vegetables, season with Papa Fike's Original Seasoning or garlic pepper. Toss to coat evenly.
4. Place each veggie on a skewer filling skewer. Grill over flame for 20-25 minutes or until tender and slightly caramelized. Make sure to rotate to even out grilling.
5. Serve as a colorful and nutritious appetizer.

NUTRITIONAL Value:
% Daily Value based on a 2000 calorie diet

Total Fat 5 g	6%
Saturated Fat 0.5 g	3%
Cholesterol 0 mg	0%
Sodium 16 mg	1%
Carbohydrates 32.2 g	12%
Dietary Fiber 4.3 g	15%
Total Sugars 4.8 g	
Protein 4.7 g	

Grumbles from the Chuckwagon:
The cowboys are howling like coyotes. It happened when I decided to liven things up. I rustled up some of these nutritious Papa Fike's veggie skewers. It's not the usual beef and beans, but gotta keep things interesting. Of course they scoffed, but after informing them I'd eat my hat if they didn't take to them. So, they got a twinkle in their eyes and plucked a skewer loaded with veggies off that hot grill and ate. And you know what? I still got my hat and a request to double the amount for next time. Woohoo!

Chrissy Hartmann

5.7 Chicken Pepper Cranberry Salad

Serving Size: 1 Tablespoon
Servings: 32
Approximate Calories: 112

Ingredients:
- 3 cups cooked chicken breast
- 1-1/2 cup Homemade Mayo (see chapter 9)
- 1 stalk of celery diced
- 1 onion diced
- 1/2 cup cranberries
- 1 teaspoon black pepper
- 1/2 cup chopped pecans

Instructions:
1. In bowl combine cooked chicken, celery, cranberries, onion, and pecans.
2. Mix together with 1 cup of homemade mayo (see chapter 9) and pepper.
3. Chill in refrigerator until needed.
4. Once chilled serve on pepper crackers.

Nutritional Value:
% Daily Value based on a 2000 calorie diet

Total Fat 6 g	8%
Saturated Fat 0.9 g	4%
Cholesterol 14 mg	5%
Sodium 113 mg	5%
Carbohydrates 3.9 g	1%
Dietary Fiber 0.2 g	1%
Total Sugars 1 g	
Protein 4 g	

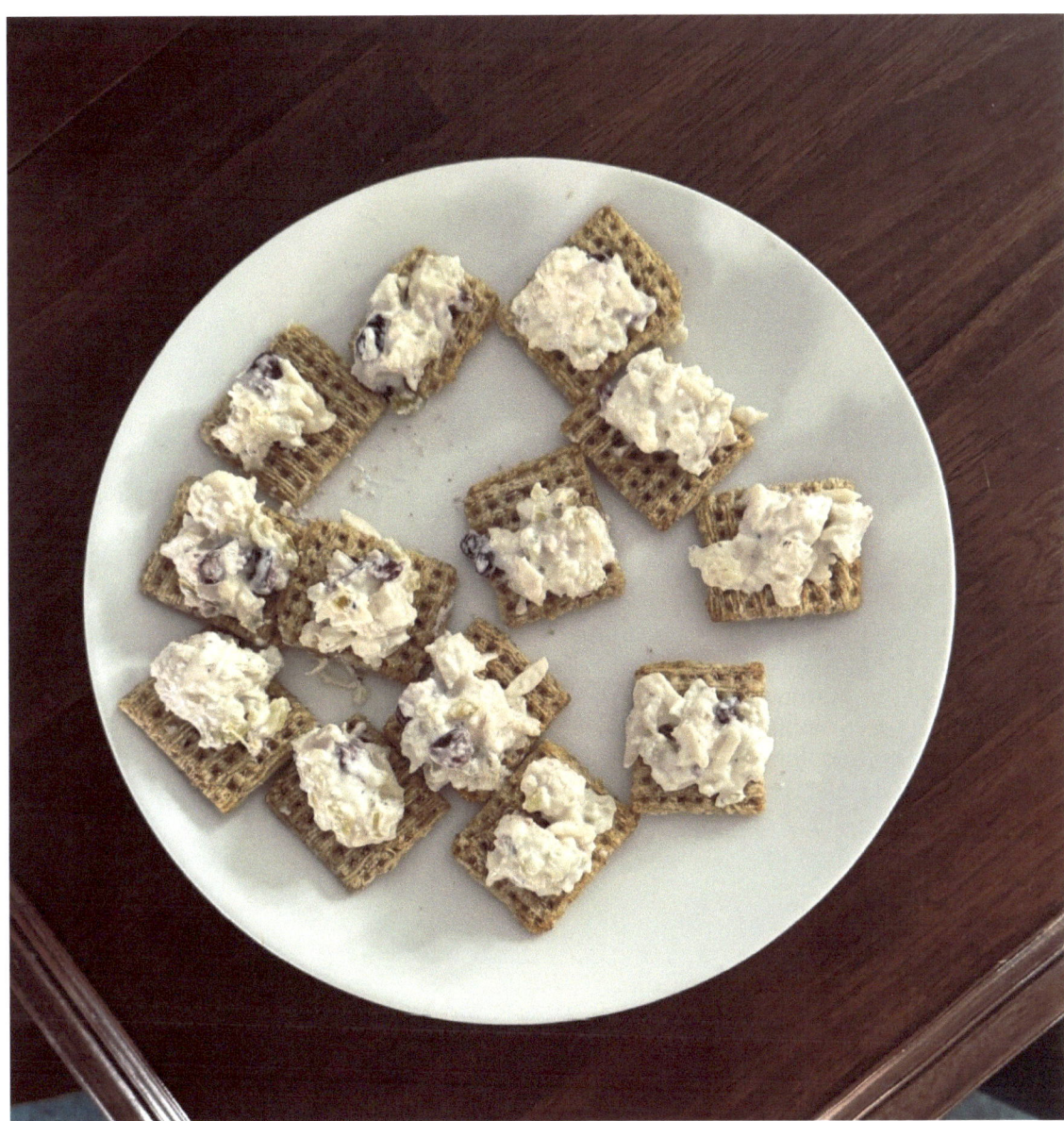

Grumbles from the Chuckwagon:
No slow rolling tumbleweed when it comes to this appetizer. Quick and easy to make. Plate up this chicken salad onto a pepper cracker and watch them disappear. A hearty treat that will keep your cowboy satisfied until the dinner bell rings.

Chrissy Hartmann

5.8 Fire Blackened Shrimp

Serving Size: 3 to 4 Shrimp
Servings: 8
Approximate Calories: 493

Ingredients:
- 1-pound large shrimp, peeled and deveined
- 1 cup buttermilk
- 1 cup cornstarch
- 2 tablespoons Papa Fike's Blackening Seasoning
- 2 tablespoons grapeseed oil
- 1/2 cup Homemade Mayo (see chapter 9)
- 2 tablespoons sweet chili sauce
- Optional: 1 tablespoon hot sauce
- 1 teaspoon honey
- 1 teaspoon garlic powder

Instructions:
1. Marinate shrimp in buttermilk for 30 minutes.
2. In a bowl mix the cornstarch and Papa Fike's blackening seasoning.
3. In a skillet (cast iron preferred) heat grapeseed oil to 350F.°
4. Dredge shrimp in cornstarch mixture, shake off any excess.
5. Fry the shrimp until golden brown, about 3 to 4 minutes.
6. In separate bowl, mix Homemade Mayo, sweet chili sauce, hot sauce, honey, and garlic powder.
7. Once done, toss them in sauce mixture until evenly coated or if preferred use as a dip.
8. Serve hot and enjoy!

Nutritional Values:
% daily value based on a 2000 calorie diet

Total Fat 30.3 g	39%
Saturated Fat 3.3 g	16%
Cholesterol 21 mg	7%
Sodium 6209 mg	270%
Carbohydrates 49.3 g	18%
Dietary Fiber 3.2 g	11%
Total Sugars 26.8 g	
Protein 6.5 g	

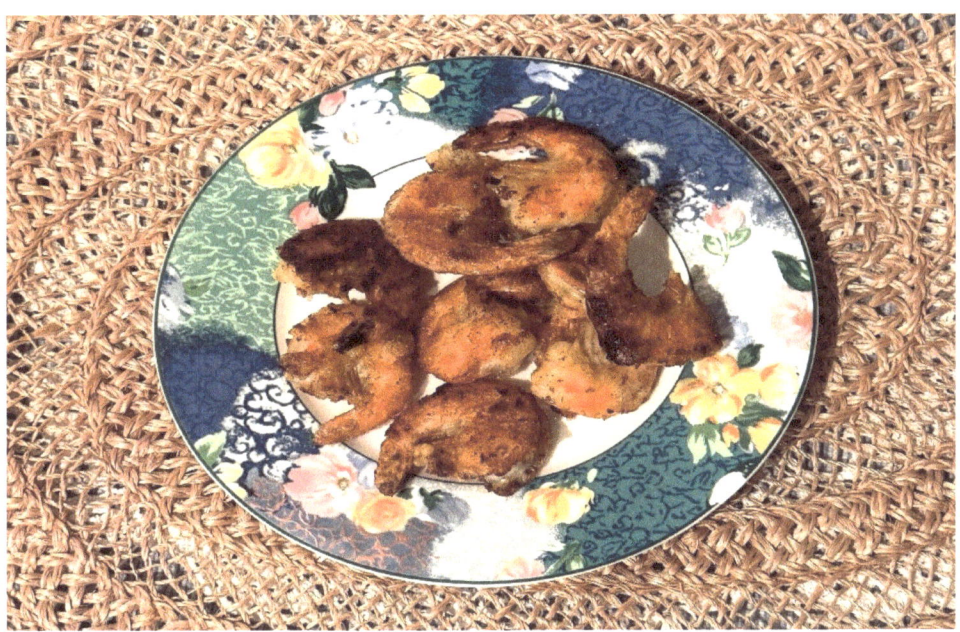

Grumbles From the Chuckwagon:
Under the vast open starry sky, I decided to cook up these here Shrimp. The cowboys stood around the campfire with bellies grumbling eager for the shrimp. With skillet in hand, I gave the cowboys fair warning they'd be hot, like branding iron hot. They just laughed at me jawing that nothing they ate would have a heat they couldn't handle. I fixed them up like the recipe and when finally plated up, they dug into the crispy shrimp. As the first bite hit, the camp echoed with hollers of a mix of surprise and delight. The fiery kick of the shrimp sauce had the toughest cowhands reaching for their canteens grinning through the spice declaring them a wild ride for their taste buds under the western moon. And with that declaration, my ticker smiled.

Chrissy Hartmann

5.9 Turkey Stuffed Mushrooms

Serving Size: 1 mushroom
Servings: 24
Approximate Calories: 117

Ingredients:
- 24 whole baby portabella mushrooms, stems removed and diced (to use later)
- 1/4 cup grapeseed oil
- 2 pounds cooked ground turkey
- 12 ounces spicy hummus
- 1/2 cup shredded sharp cheddar cheese
- Optional: 1/2 cup zesty Vidalia sauce (See chapter 9 for recipe)

Instructions:
1. Preheat oven to 375°F.
2. In a bowl, combine cooked ground turkey, spicy hummus (see chapter 5), diced mushroom stems, breadcrumbs, and grapeseed oil.
3. Add 1/2 teaspoon of Vidalia sauce to bottom of each mushroom (see chapter 9)
4. Fill each mushroom cap with hummus ground turkey mixture.
5. Place each mushroom into a 9×13 baking dish.
6. Cover with aluminum foil and bake in preheated oven for 15-20 minutes or until mushrooms are tender.
7. Remove from oven, uncover, and sprinkle cheddar cheese on top of mushrooms. Place aluminum foil back on until ready to eat.
8. Serve and enjoy.

Nutrition Value:
% daily value based on a 2000 calorie diet

Total Fat 7.4 g	10%
Saturated Fat 1.4 g	7%
Cholesterol 11 mg	4%
Sodium 211 mg	9%
Carbohydrates 7.2 g	3%
Dietary Fiber 3 g	11%
Total Sugars 0 g	
Protein 6.8 g	

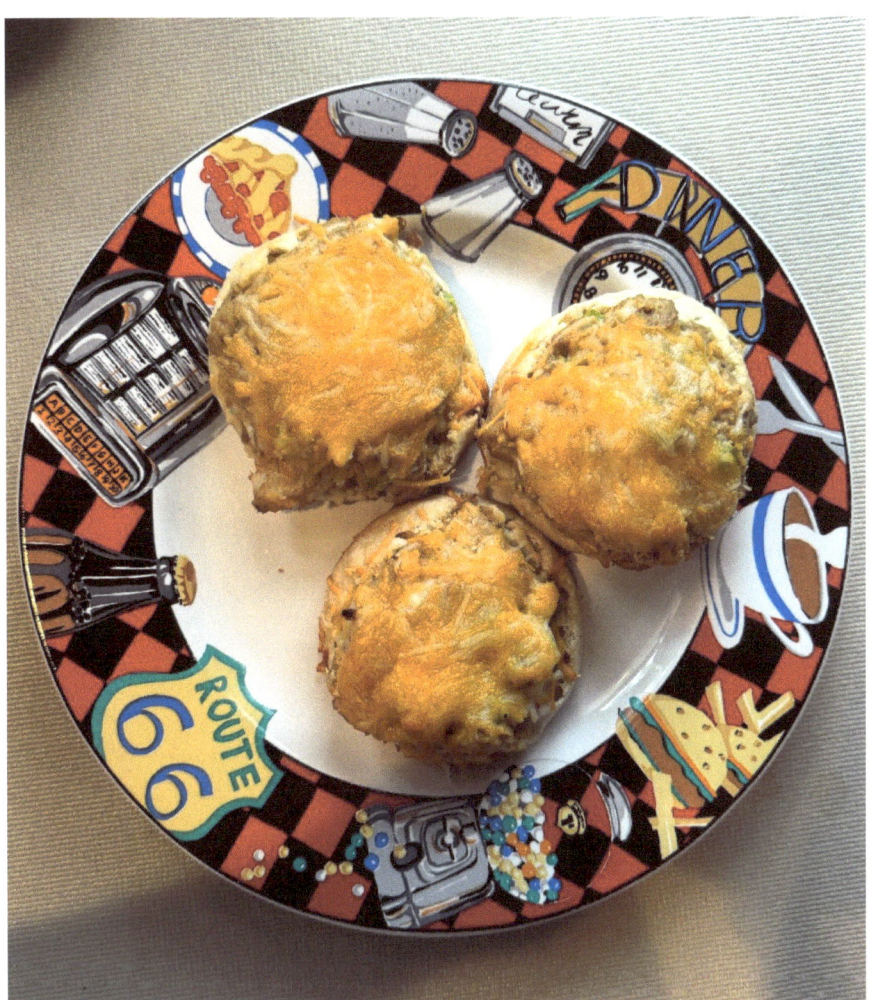

Grumbles from the Chuckwagon:
There gone in 8 seconds flat. These turkey Stuffed Mushrooms are a triumph of flavor at the chuckwagon. A burst of savory goodness in every bite, they're a perfect dish for hungry cowboys. The grapeseed oil not only adds a touch of richness but also keeps these morsels tender and mouthwatering. One bite, and you'll be sending out the posse for more.

Chrissy Hartmann

5.10 Plum Delicious Fried Greenies

Serving Size: 1/3 cup
Servings: 6
Approximate Calories: 534

Ingredients:
- 1-pound green beans, trimmed
- ⅓ cup all-purpose flour
- 3 tablespoons cornstarch
- 1 large egg
- ⅓ cup club soda, cold
- 2 cups grapeseed oil
- ¼ teaspoon Himalayan salt
- 1/2 teaspoon garlic pepper
- Plum sauce with ginger for dipping (See chapter 9)

Instructions:
1. Heat grapeseed oil to 375 degrees Fahrenheit in large saucepan.
2. Wash and trim ends of the green beans.
3. In medium-sized bowl, whisk flour and cornstarch together.
4. In another bowl, beat the egg then stir in club soda.
5. Add liquid mixture to flour mixture then whisk to combine.
6. Dip each green bean in batter, place in pot of grapeseed oil, cook 3-4 minutes until golden.
7. Remove from oil, transfer to paper towels on plate. Repeat until all green beans are cooked.
8. Season with salt and pepper. Serve with plum sauce with ginger.

Nutritional Value:
% daily value based on a 2000 calorie diet
Total Fat 35.1 g 45%
Saturated Fat 3.7 g 19%
Cholesterol 62 mg 21%
Carbohydrates 51.2 g 19%
Sodium 30 mg 1%
Protein: 3.1 g
Fiber 1.2 g 4%
Total Sugar 0.4 g
Potassium 65 mg 1%

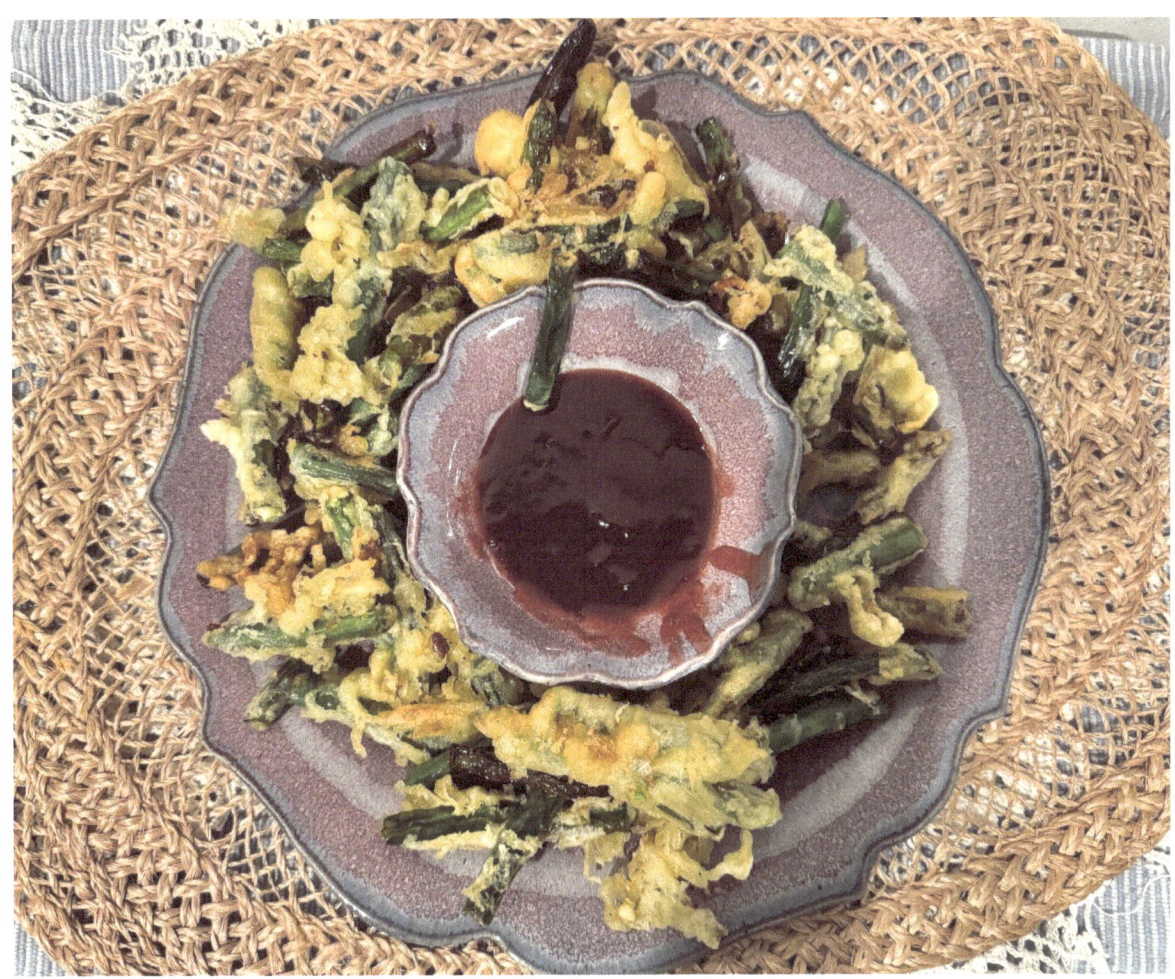

Grumbles from the Chuckwagon:

I slapped the basket of fried green beans onto the table, dusted off my hands, and gave a holler. "Come and get it, boys!" They ambled over, squinting at the basket like it held rattlesnakes instead of something to tide them over until supper was ready.
"Fried green beans?" one muttered, raising an eyebrow.
"Best give it a try," I said, nodding to the bowl of plum sauce beside it. "Dip 'em." The first cowboy bit down, and his eyes widened. The others followed, crunching through the crispy coating, that sweet plum tang catching 'em by surprise. "Gus," one said, grinning, "you're gonna spoil us if you keep this up."

Chrissy Hartmann

5.11 Cauliflower Cow Patties

Serving Size: 2 patties
Servings: 2
Approximate Calories: 252

Ingredients:
- 1 head cauliflower (3 cups)
- ¾ cups almond flour
- 1 egg
- 1 teaspoon garlic pepper
- 1 teaspoon chipotle seasoning
- 2 tablespoons grapeseed oil

Instructions:
1. Chop cauliflower into tiny florets.
2. Boil cauliflower until soft.
3. Mix in medium bowl almond flour, garlic pepper, salt, egg, and chipotle seasoning while cauliflower cooks.
4. Add cauliflower to mixture.
5. Using 2 tablespoons of cauliflower mixture, form into ¼ inch patties.
6. Heat skillet with half of grapeseed oil on low heat, once hot, cook patties for 6-8 minutes on each side using the rest of grapeseed oil as you go until golden brown.
7. Serve hot with lemon dipping sauce (see chapter 9) with meal.

Nutritional Values:
% daily value based on a 2000 calorie diet

Total Fat 25 g	37 %
Saturated Fat 4 g	18%
Cholesterol 23 mg	14%
Sodium 376 mg	25 %
Carbohydrates 12 g	5%
Dietary Fiber 5.34 g	22%
Total Sugars 2 g	
Protein 11 g	

Grumbles from the Chuckwagon:
Well, I tell ya, these young cowpokes took one look at my cauliflower cow patties and swore up and down they were "cow patties" fresh outta the field, I'd say with a shake of my head. Had to near threaten all of them just to get them to take a bite, and wouldn't ya know, soon as they did, their chomping down like it's prime rib. Guess they learned quick—don't question the cook if ya want a good meal.

5.12 Chipotle Chicken Wings

Serving Size: 5-6
Servings: 6
Approximate Calories: 269

Ingredients:
- 2 pounds chicken wings, drumettes and flats
- 2 tablespoons grapeseed oil
- 2 teaspoons garlic pepper
- 1 teaspoon salt
- 1 teaspoon onion powder
- optional: ½ teaspoon chipotle chili powder

Instructions:
1. Preheat air fryer to 400 °F for 5 minutes.
2. Prepare wings, pat dry
3. In plastic bag, mix grapeseed oil and wings.
4. Sprinkle garlic pepper, onion powder, salt, and chipotle chili powder seasonings over wings, shake closed bag.
5. Remove from plastic bag, place in fryer, one level. Air fry 25 to 30 minutes, shake half-way through.
6. Remove from air fryer, serve with celery, ranch or blue cheese.

Nutritional Value:
% daily value based on a 2000 calorie diet
Total Fat 19.3 g 25%
Saturated Fat 2.3 g 12%
Cholesterol 30 mg 10%
Sodium 6493 mg 283%
Carbohydrates 13.5 g 5%
Fiber 1 g 3%
Total Sugar 5.9 g
Protein 19.3 g

Grumbles from the Chuckwagon:
I wiped my brow, eyeing the wings. "You fellas think you're real clever, asking for wings after a long day, huh?" I grumbled, grabbing the grapeseed oil and spices. "Back in my day, beans and sourdough did the trick, but fine, I'll make your fancy chicken wings." The smell of crispy, golden wings had 'em crowding around, hats in hand, and I couldn't help but laugh. "Can't believe y'all needed wings tonight," I muttered, passing out the first batch.

Chrissy Hartmann

The Grub Wrangler's Wisdom:

Chapter 6 Main Course Marvels

Howdy, famished cowpoke! Welcome to "Main Course Marvels," where we'll be cooking up western feasts that'll make your belly sing like a campfire serenade.

Now, what's our secret ingredient for these marvels?
Well shoot, I'm sure you know by now, but it's none other than grapeseed oil – the culinary wrangler's best friend. Whether it's BBQ chicken with a smoky twang, tuna melts that'll make your taste buds two-step, or fried catfish that's a riverbank revelation, grapeseed oil is our choice.

Why grapeseed oil, you ask? Well, it's the unsung hero in the chuckwagon, with a high smoke point that keeps the sizzle without the fizzle. Plus, it packs a punch of antioxidants, giving these here main dishes of grub a health boost without stampeding over the flavor.

Now, lean in for a chuckle from the riverbanks. My bestie, bless her adventurous soul, took me fishing for the first time. She landed a catfish so big, folks started wondering if those whiskered critters were secretly man-eaters. Meanwhile, I ended up wrangling an old boot instead of a fish. Turns out, my bestie had a knack for hooking big ones, and I was left pondering the dangers of the elusive man-eating catfish!

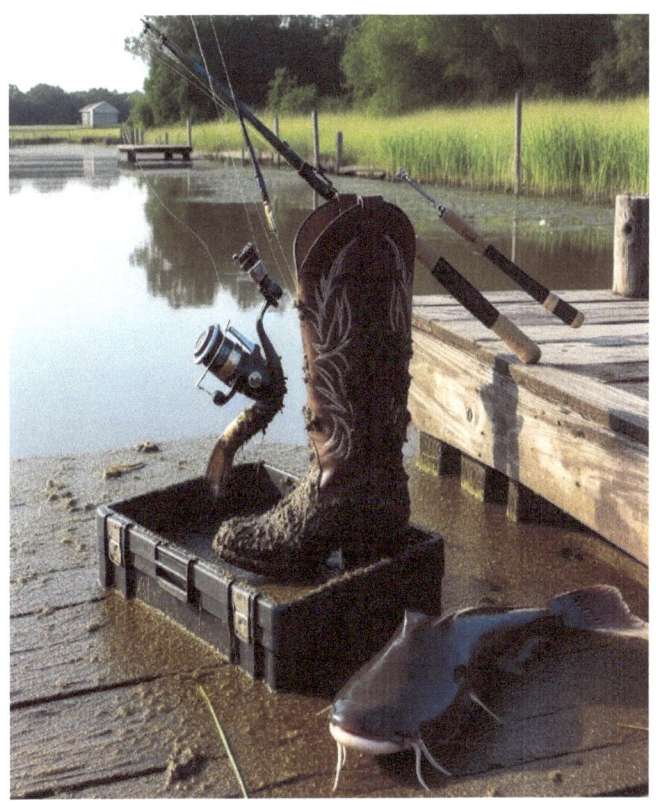

So, pull those boots on flavor trailblazers! Let's rustle up some main course marvels and turn your table into a taste adventure with a side of wild catfish tales. And hey partner, if you're missing a fishing boot, I know where to find it.

Chrissy Hartmann

6.1 Blackened Catfish with Lemon Cream Sauce

Serving Size: 1 filet
Servings: 4
Approximate Calories: 452

Ingredients:
For the Catfish:
- 4 catfish fillets
- 2 tablespoons grapeseed oil (for frying)
- 4 tablespoons Papa Fike's Blackened Seasoning
- Salt and pepper to taste

For the Lemon Cream Sauce:
- 1 tablespoon grapeseed oil (for sauce)
- 2 tablespoons butter
- 1 cup heavy cream
- Zest and juice of 1 lemon
- 4 tablespoons dry vermouth
- Salt and pepper to taste
- Optional: 1 garlic clove, minced
- Optional: 1 tablespoon chopped fresh parsley, garnish

Instructions:
1. In a saucepan, heat 1 tablespoon grapeseed oil and butter over medium heat.
2. Add minced garlic and sauté until fragrant, about 30 seconds.
3. Stir in cream, lemon zest, lemon juice, and dry vermouth.
4. - Simmer sauce for 3-5 minutes, stirring occasionally, until it thickens slightly.
5. Season with salt and pepper to taste.

6. Now that lemon sauce is ready, prepare Catfish. Rub catfish fillets generously with blackened seasoning, salt, and pepper.
7. Heat 2 tablespoons of grapeseed oil in a cast-iron skillet over medium-high heat.
8. Fry each fillet for 3-4 minutes on each side, until blackened and crispy on the outside, and flaky inside. Remove and plate.
9. Drizzle Lemon Cream Sauce over catfish. Garnish with fresh parsley. Serve with steamed green beans and red potatoes.

Nutrition Values:
% daily value based on a 2000 calorie diet
Total Fat 82 g   105%
Saturated Fat 33.2 g   166%
Cholesterol 198 mg   66%
Sodium 583 mg   25%
Carbohydrates 20.1 g   7%
Dietary Fiber 1.9 g   7%
Total Sugars 1g
Protein 21.1 g

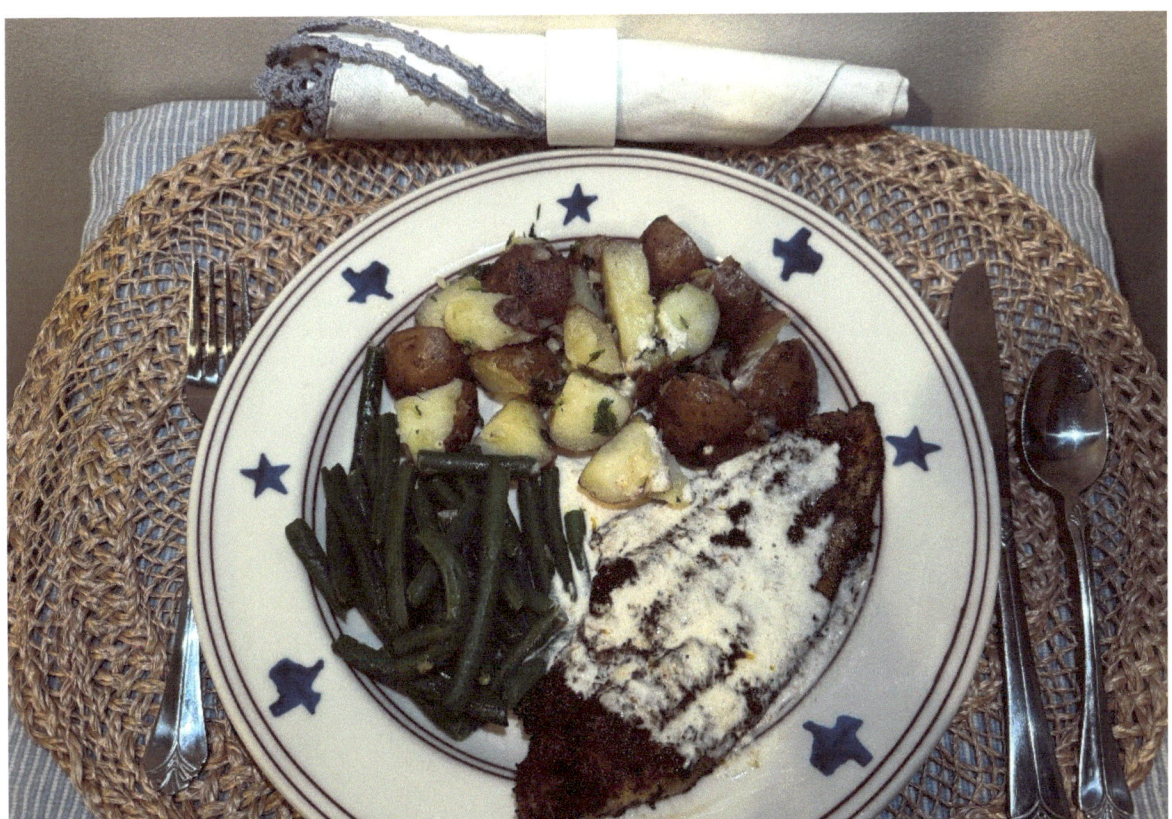

Chrissy Hartmann

6.2 Zesty Lemon Chicken

Serving Size: 1 bowl
Servings: 4
Approximate Calories: 140

Ingredients:
- 4 boneless, skinless chicken breasts
- 2 tablespoons grapeseed oil
- 2 cloves garlic, minced
- Zest and juice of 1 lemon
- Papa Fike's Original Seasoning
- 4 Cups cooked wild rice

Instructions:
1. Season chicken breasts with Papa Fike's Original Seasoning.
2. In skillet, heat grapeseed oil over medium-high heat.
3. Add minced garlic and sauté briefly.
4. Place chicken in skillet and cook until browned and cooked through.
5. Drizzle lemon juice and zest over chicken before serving It over a bed of cooked wild rice

Nutritional Value:
% Daily Value based on a 2000 calorie diet

Total Fat	4.1 g	5%
Saturated Fat	0.6 g	3%
Cholesterol	11 mg	4%
Sodium	13 mg	1%
Carbohydrates	18.9 g	7%
Dietary Fiber	0.4 g	1%
Total Sugars	0.4 g	
Protein	5.9 g	

Grumbles from the Chuckwagon:
Tipping our hat to Papa Fike's Original Seasoning – the unsung hero that's been quietly enhancing flavors. Not one to seek the spotlight, but we here at chuckwagon central believe it's high time Papa Fike makes its zest known. Sure, we're all about the grapeseed, but this is one seasoning we must throw the spotlight on. If it weren't for its flavor taking center stage in our Zesty Lemon Chicken dish, our chuckwagon might as well be serving up tumbleweeds.

6.3 Chipotle Shrimp Scampi

Serving Size: 3-5 shrimp
Servings: 4
Approximate Calories: 167

Ingredients:
- 1-pound large shrimp, peeled and deveined
- 2 tablespoons grapeseed oil
- 2 tablespoon chipotle seasoning
- 2 cloves garlic, minced
- Zest and juice of 1 lemon
- 1/4 cup white wine

Instructions:
1. In bowl, season shrimp with chipotle seasoning, and lemon zest.
2. Heat grapeseed oil in skillet over medium-high heat.
3. Add minced garlic and sauté briefly.
4. Add shrimp and cook until they turn pink (about 2 minutes).
5. Pour in white wine and lemon juice. Simmer until thickens.
6. Garnish with fresh parsley and serve over pasta or with crusty bread.

Nutritional Values:
% Daily Value Based on a 2000 calorie diet

Total Fat 6.8 g	9%
Saturated Fat 0.7 g	3%
Cholesterol 162 mg	54%
Sodium 143 mg	6%
Carbohydrates 3.2 g	1%
Dietary Fiber 0.1 g	0%
Total Sugars 0.1 g	
Protein 21.4 g	

Grumbles from the Chuckwagon:
My cowgirl's heart might have hit a bump in the trail, but it don't mean giving up the good grub. And Chipotle Shrimp Scampi cooked in grapeseed oil is our secret to keeping things light and heart friendly. Even after a showdown with that old heart attack, she's still savoring the joys of a good meal – zesty chipotle shrimp scampi done right with grapeseed oil. Yeehaw!

Chrissy Hartmann

6.4 Spirited Beef Stir-Fry

Serving Size: 1 cup
Servings: 4
Approximate Calories: 633

Ingredients:
- 8 ounces flank steak (cut in narrow strips)
- 1 Cup bell peppers
- 1 Cup broccoli
- 1/2 Cup carrots, diced
- 1 Cup snap peas
- 1 Cup cauliflower
- 1 Can water chestnuts, sliced
- 2 tablespoons cornstarch
- 2 tablespoons red pepper flakes
- 2 tablespoons grapeseed oil
- 2 cloves garlic, minced
- 1/4 cup soy sauce
- 1 tablespoon honey
- 4 Cups cooked wild rice

Instructions:
1. Cut vegetables into bite-sized pieces.
2. Toss flank steak strips in cornstarch
3. Heat grapeseed oil in a large skillet.
4. Add flank steak strips, minced garlic and stir.
5. Add vegetables and stir-fry until tender, but still crisp.
6. In small bowl, mix soy sauce and honey, pour over beef and vegetables, stir until thickens.
7. Serve over rice.

Nutritional Value:
% Daily Value based on a 2000 calorie diet

Total Fat 10.6 g	14%
Saturated Fat 1.3 g	7%
Cholesterol 0 mg	0%
Sodium 927 mg	40%
Carbohydrates 167.8 g	61%
Dietary Fiber 7.1 g	25%
Total Sugars 11.5 g	
Protein 18.7g	

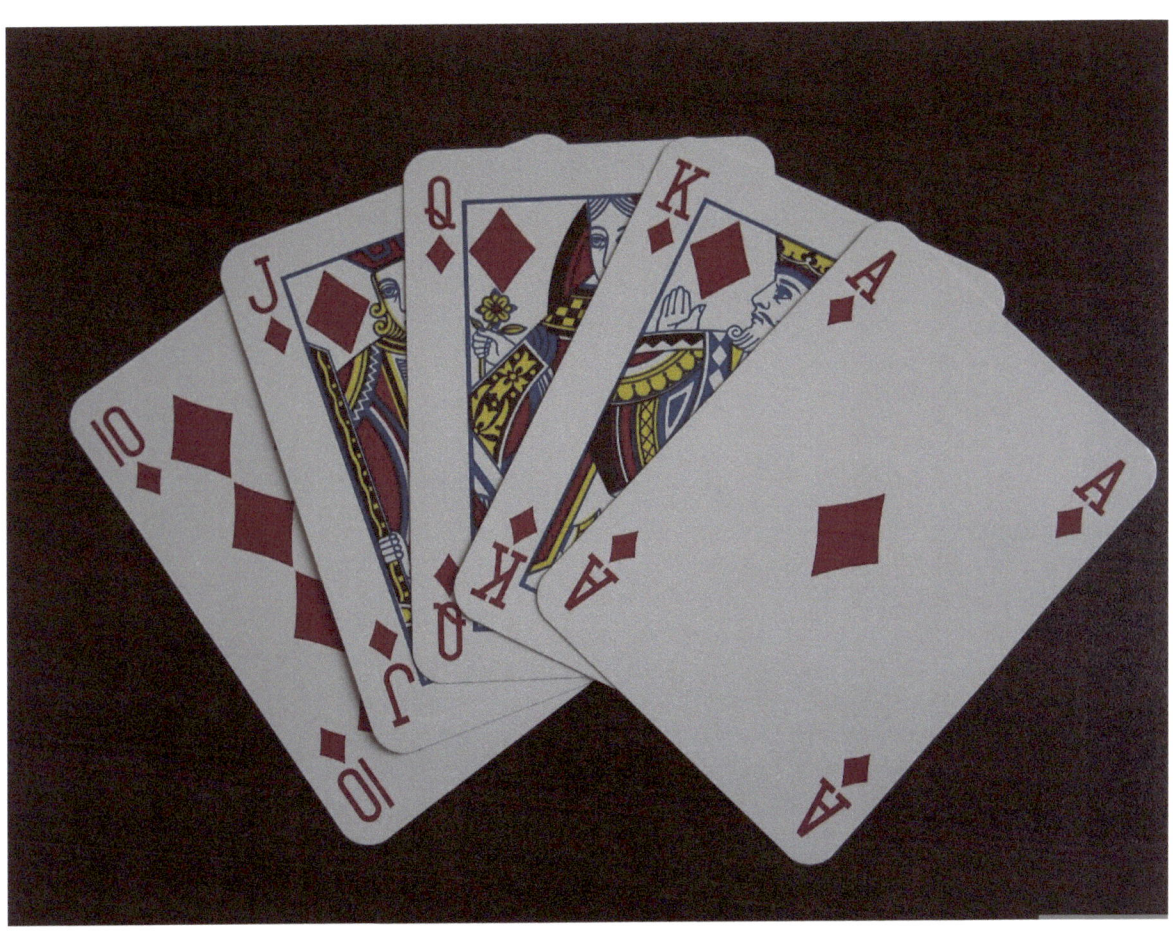

Grumbles from the Chuckwagon:
When I'm out for a night of poker and the chuckwagon is quiet, my cowgirl turns to a taste of excitement in the kitchen. It's quick as prairie wind tossing veggies and sizzling beef, faster than a herd of wild mustangs. She insists the flavors dance like a hoedown in her mouth and it's a party dish that'll keeps her going until I ride back at sunrise. So, if the ranch feels a bit lonesome, beef stir fry just might be the yeehaw your taste buds are craving.

Chrissy Hartmann

6.5 Woodland Mushroom Risotto

Serving Size: 1 cup
Servings: 8
Approximate Calories: 366

Ingredients:
- 1-1/2 cups Arborio rice
- 8 cups vegetable or chicken broth
- 1 cup white wine
- 2 tablespoons grapeseed oi
- 1 cup mushrooms, sliced
- 1/4 cup grated Parmesan cheese
- Salt and pepper to taste

Instructions:
1. In large saucepan, heat grapeseed oil.
2. Add sliced mushrooms and sauté until browned.
3. Stir in Arborio rice and cook for a few minutes.
4. Pour in white wine and cook until it's mostly absorbed.
5. Gradually add hot broth, one ladle at a time, stirring until rice is creamy and tender.
6. Stir in Parmesan cheese and season with salt and pepper.
7. Serve hot with a crusty bread.

Nutritional Value:
% Daily Value based on a 2000 calorie diet

Total Fat 10.2 g	13%
Saturated Fat 1.7 g	9%
Cholesterol 1 mg	0%
Sodium 1550 mg	67%
Carbohydrates 41.8 g	15%
Dietary Fiber 1.5 g	5%
Total Sugars 2.2 g	
Protein 14 g	

Grumbles from the Chuckwagon:
Here's another dish my cowgirl's heart hankers for because it's comfort in a bowl just like a well-worn saddle. Whip it up in your chuckwagon– simmering rice, savory mushrooms, and a splash of broth. The creamy richness is like a sunset over the mesa, and it fills your belly with warmth. So, when the day's been a rough ride, mushroom risotto is my cowgirl's campfire for the soul.

6.6 Pecan Berry Chicken

Serving Size: 1/2 cup
Servings: 8
Approximate Calories: 242

Ingredients:
- 4 cups boneless chicken, cubed
- 2 Tablespoons grapeseed oil
- 1 cup raspberries
- 1 cup blueberries
- 1/2 cup pecans
- shredded Lettuce

Instructions:
1. Heat grapeseed oil in skillet.
2. Add chicken to skillet and cook over medium heat for about 7 minutes.
3. Add the pecans to skillet until toasted.
4. Place the chicken and pecans over bed of shredded lettuce.
5. Sprinkle raspberries and blueberries over top the chicken, pecans, and lettuce.

Nutritional Value:
% Daily Value based on a 2000 calorie diet

Total Fat 15.2 g	19%
Saturated Fat 1.7 g	8%
Cholesterol 54 mg	18%
Sodium 44 mg	2%
Carbohydrates 7 g	3%
Dietary Fiber 2.4 g	9%
Total Sugars 3 g	
Protein 21.6 g	

Grumbles from the Chuckwagon:
These here cowboys' hearts are as wild as the west and their taste buds are no different. Grilled chicken with pecans, berries over a bed of lettuce is grub they love. It's a symphony of flavors that sing like a campfire under the stars. The grilled chicken dances with the crunch of pecans and the berries add a sweet kick. Like a moonlit serenade, it's a wholesome roundup that satisfies their appetite while making those taste buds do a hoedown.

Chrissy Hartmann

6.7 Pork Tenderloin with Apple Compote

Serving Size 6 ounces
Servings: 4
Approximate Calories: 282

Ingredients:
- 1 pork tenderloin
- 2 tablespoons grapeseed oil
- 2 apples, peeled and sliced
- 1/4 cup brown sugar
- 1/4 cup apple cider
- 1/2 teaspoon cinnamon
- Salt and pepper to taste

Instructions:
1. Preheat oven to 350°F.
2. Season pork tenderloin with salt and pepper.
3. Heat grapeseed oil in oven-safe skillet and Sear pork on all sides until browned.
4. Transfer skillet to oven and roast for about 20 minutes.
5. Meanwhile, in separate skillet, cook apples with brown sugar, apple cider, and cinnamon until they form compote.
6. Slice the pork and serve with apple compote.

Nutritional Value:
% Daily Value based on a 2000 calorie diet

Total Fat 10 g	13%
Saturated Fat 1.7 g	8%
Cholesterol 62 mg	21%
Sodium 52 mg	2%
Carbohydrates 26.3 g	10%
Dietary Fiber 2.9 g	10%
Total Sugars 22.1 g	
Protein 22.6 g	

Grumbles from the Chuckwagon:
Now, I ain't one for mush, but if you all try my pork tenderloin with apple compote, expect love notes from the cowhands. Found one in my apron last week. Consider this your warning, this dish ain't just for eating. And hey, boys, my gal don't take to kindly to someone leaving heart notes in my apron. Stop!

6.8 Christmas Spinach Chicken

Serving Size: 1 chicken breast
Servings: 4
Approximate Calories: 859

Ingredients:
- 4 Chicken breasts, diced.
- 3 tablespoons grapeseed oil
- 1/4 teaspoon lemon pepper
- 8 ounces fresh spinach, washed and chopped.
- 2 Roma tomatoes
- 4 Cups cooked white rice

Instructions:
1. In skillet heat up grapeseed oil.
2. Add diced chicken and lemon pepper to skillet and cook until done.
3. On plate, place 1 cup cooked white rice.
4. Layer spinach, tomato slice, and chicken on top of rice.
5. Serve with crusted bread. Enjoy!

Nutritional Value:
% Daily Value based on a 2000 calorie diet

Total Fat 14.5 g	19%
Saturated Fat 2.1 g	11%
Cholesterol 32 mg	11%
Sodium 88 mg	4%
Carbohydrates 152.4 g	55%
Dietary Fiber 4.4 g	16%
Total Sugars 2.1 g	
Protein 25.9 g	

Grumbles from the Chuckwagon:
My gal thinks I oughta slap on a Santa hat while I'm cooking this Christmas chicken with rice, like I'm some jolly fool. I told her, "Ain't no way I'm playing dress-up while I'm feeding cowboys." Hmm? Maybe later though. Ho Ho Ho!

Chrissy Hartmann

6.9 Rodeo Peppered Beef

Serving Size: 1/2 cup
Servings: 8
Approximate Calories: 400

Ingredients:
- 2-pound round beef roast
- 1 can cola
- 6 ounces beef broth
- 3 tablespoon grapeseed oil
- 1/2 cup water
- 3 tablespoons flour
- garlic pepper to taste
- Cooked wild rice or noodles

Instructions:
1. In small bowl mix together water and flour, stir out lumps.
2. Rub grapeseed oil and garlic pepper into beef roast.
3. In crockpot pour cola and beef broth in.
4. Place beef roast in crockpot and cook for 5 hours on medium heat. Shred after 3 hours.
5. After 3 hours, pour in water flour mixture to thicken broth.
6. Serve with your choice of wild rice or noodles.
7. Plate with glazed carrots. Enjoy!

Nutritional Values:
% Daily Value for a 2000 calorie diet

Total Fat 11.1 g	14%
Saturated Fat 2.6 g	13%
Cholesterol 76 mg	25%
Sodium 130 mg	6%
Carbohydrates 41. 7g	15%
Dietary Fiber 3 g	11%
Total Sugars 5.4 g	
Protein 33.1 g	

Grumbles from the Chuckwagon:
If your chuckwagon has an outlet, then fire up your crockpot. Here's one recipe that cooks faster than a tumbleweed rolling across the open range. Preparing this meal is easier than cleaning my six-shooter. The crockpot cooking your chow will give you just enough time to do your evening chores before the flavors of that first bite explodes in your mouth like the stars over the Texas sky.

6.10 Chipotle Steak Taco

Serving Size: 1
Servings: 4
Approximate Calories: 283

Ingredients:
- 1-pound top sirloin strips
- 1+ tablespoons Chipotle Seasoning
- 2 tablespoons grapeseed oil
- 2 tomatoes, diced
- 1 green pepper, diced
- 1 cup shredded Tex-Mex cheese
- 1 sweet onion
- 2 cups lettuce
- 4 corn street taco shells

Instructions:
1. Cut steak strips into strips and marinate in chipotle seasoning.
2. Heat skillet with grapeseed oil and seer steak until cooked.
3. Prepare corn taco shells.
4. Stuff taco shells with lettuce, steak, tomato, onion, green pepper, and cheese.
5. Serve with sour cream, tortilla chips and mango avocado salsa.

Nutritional Value:
% daily value based on a 2000 calorie diet

Total Fat 22.1 g	28%
Saturated Fat 4.1 g	20%
Cholesterol 193 mg	64%
Sodium 154 mg	7%
Carbohydrates 17.6 g	3%
Dietary Fiber 0.8 g	3%
Total Sugars 0.9 g	
Protein 8.7 g	

Grumbles from the Chuckwagon:
When these here steak tacos hit the chow menu, it's like a cattle stampede at sunset. The cowboys rise faster than the rooster crows for a shot at these here chipotle taco delights. the promise of them steak tacos turns tired eyes into young sprouts. The chuck wagon becomes a dinner battleground, and by sunset , plates are piled high with flavors that make tomorrow's hardships feel a world away.

Chrissy Hartmann

6.11 Sundance Tuna Melts

Serving Size: 6 ounces
Servings: 6 to 8
Approximate Calories: 307

Ingredients:
- 2 cans, 5 ounces each white tuna, drained
- 1/4 Cup Homemade Mayo (See chapter 9 for recipe)
- 1 cup diced onion
- 1 tablespoon chipotle powder
- 1 cup honey mustard
- 1 celery stalk
- 2 English muffins
- salt and pepper to taste
- 1 cup shredded sharp cheddar cheese
- Optional: Pickles for garnish

Instructions:
1. **Preheat** oven broiler to 350 °F.
2. In bowl mix tuna, Homemade Mayo (see chapter 9), onion, celery, chipotle powder, Dijon mustard, salt, and pepper until evenly combined.
3. Slice English muffins in half, place on baking sheet.
4. Spread tuna mixture onto each English muffin.
5. Sprinkle shredded sharp cheddar cheese on top of tuna mixture.
6. Place baking sheet under broiler for 8-10 minutes or until cheese is bubbly.
7. Remove and serve immediately with pickles and kale chips.

Nutritional Value:
% Daily Value based on a 2000 calorie diet

Total Fat 13.6 g	17%
Saturated Fat 6.7 g	34%
Cholesterol 58 mg	19%
Sodium 755 mg	33%
Carbohydrates 16.6 g	6%
Dietary Fiber 2.4 g	9%
Total Sugars 2.1 g	
Protein 32.8 g	

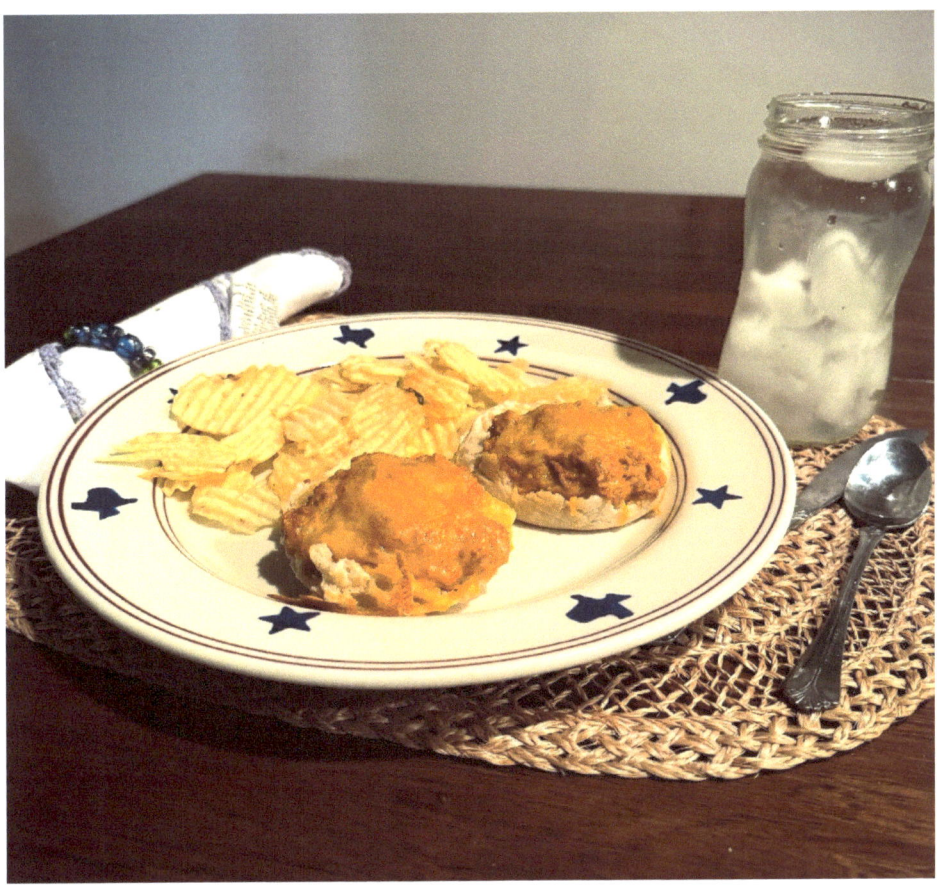

Grumbles from the Chuckwagon:
When the cowhands are hungry and their bellies are growling, I pull out this wild card. They are quick to make like a rattle snake strike. These tuna melts have a sunburst of flavor that will dance across the taste buds. As soon as they finish one, they're howling for more like a pack of coyotes. Serve them up with pickles and kale chips and your chuckwagon won't ever be empty.

Chrissy Hartmann

6.12 Rustler's Beef Stew

Serving Size: 1 bowl
Servings: 4
Approximate Calories: 498

Ingredients:
- 2 pounds beef stew meat
- 2 tablespoons grapeseed oil
- 4 cups beef broth
- 1 1/2 teaspoons flour (to thicken broth)
- 1 onion, diced
- 4 carrots, sliced
- 4 potatoes, diced
- 1 cup peas
- 1 cup cut green beans
- 2 cloves garlic, minced
- 2 stalks celery, diced
- 1-1/2 tablespoons Papa Fike's original seasoning

Instructions:
1. Coat meat lightly with 1 1/2 teaspoons of flour (Roux method).
2. In a large Dutch oven, heat grapeseed oil over medium-high heat. Brown the beef stew meat.
3. Add diced onion and minced garlic, sautéing until softened.
4. Pour in beef broth, add carrots, potatoes, peas, green beans, celery, Papa Fike's Original seasoning.
5. Bring stew to a boil, then reduce heat and simmer for 1.5 to 2 hours until meat is tender.
6. Serve with crusty bread.

Nutritional Facts:
% daily value based on a 2000 calorie diet

Total Fat 28.2 g	36%
Saturated Fat 3.5 g	17%
Cholesterol 22 mg	7%
Sodium 226 mg	10%
Carbohydrates 47.4 g	17%
Dietary Fiber 9.4 g	3%
Total Sugars 5.1 g	
Protein 15.6 g	

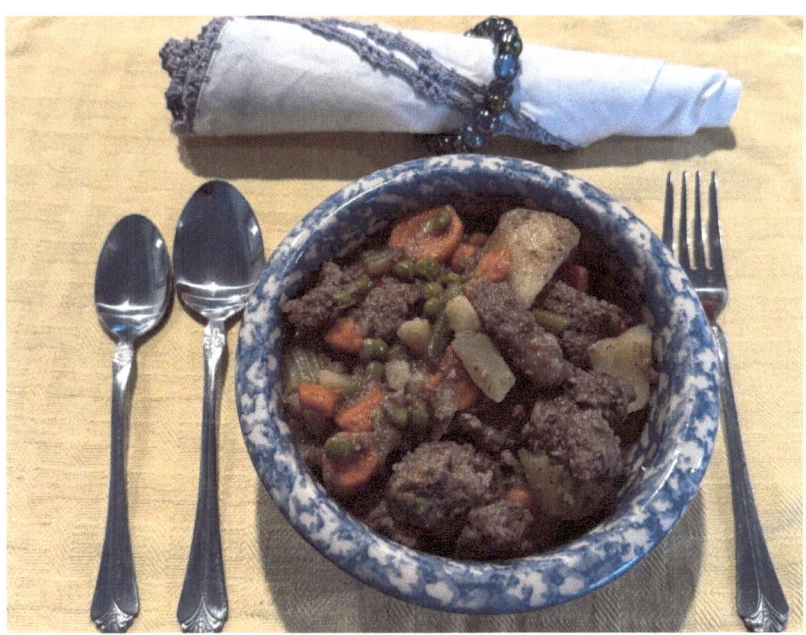

Grumbles from the Chuckwagon:
This here hardy beef stew will keep you going on the long trail rides. It's packed with meat, taters, and veggies galore, all the eats a cowboy loves. So, fill his belly and he'll be sure to thank you afterwards. Heck, some of us around the chuckwagon have even received a kiss or two for this meal, but I'll never tell who's branding those kisses. Yuck!

Chrissy Hartmann

6.13 Chicken Soft Taco

Serving Size: 1 soft taco
Servings: 4
Approximate Calories: 374

Ingredients:
- 1/2 pounds chicken breasts cut into bite size pieces
- 1 tablespoon chili powder
- 1 teaspoon cumin
- 1/4 teaspoon oregano
- 1/4 teaspoon pepper
- 2 tablespoons apple cider vinegar
- 4 tablespoons grapeseed oil divided
- 2 bell peppers sliced
- 1/2 large red onion sliced
- 4 flour tortilla shells

INSTRUCTIONS
1. Combine chicken, chili powder, cumin, oregano, salt, pepper, vinegar, and 1 tablespoon grapeseed oil and marinate for 30 minutes.
2. Heat 1 tablespoon of grapeseed oil in a large skillet over medium-high heat. Sauté chicken pieces for 8-10 minutes until golden brown and cooked through. Remove chicken from pan.
3. In same pan, add in 2 tablespoons grapeseed oil, peppers, and onion. Sauté for 5-6 minutes until softened and caramelized.
4. Place tortillas on plates, top with chicken, cheese, and veggies. Roll and wrap ends.
5. Serve with salsa, sour cream, guacamole, or pico.

Nutritional Value:
% Daily Value based on a 2000 calorie diet

Total Fat 19 g	24%
Saturated Fat 2.7 g	13%
Cholesterol 50 mg	17%
Sodium 80 m g	3%
Carbohydrates 12.7 g	5%
Dietary Fiber 2.4 g	8%
Total Sugars 0.4 g	
Protein 18.2 g	

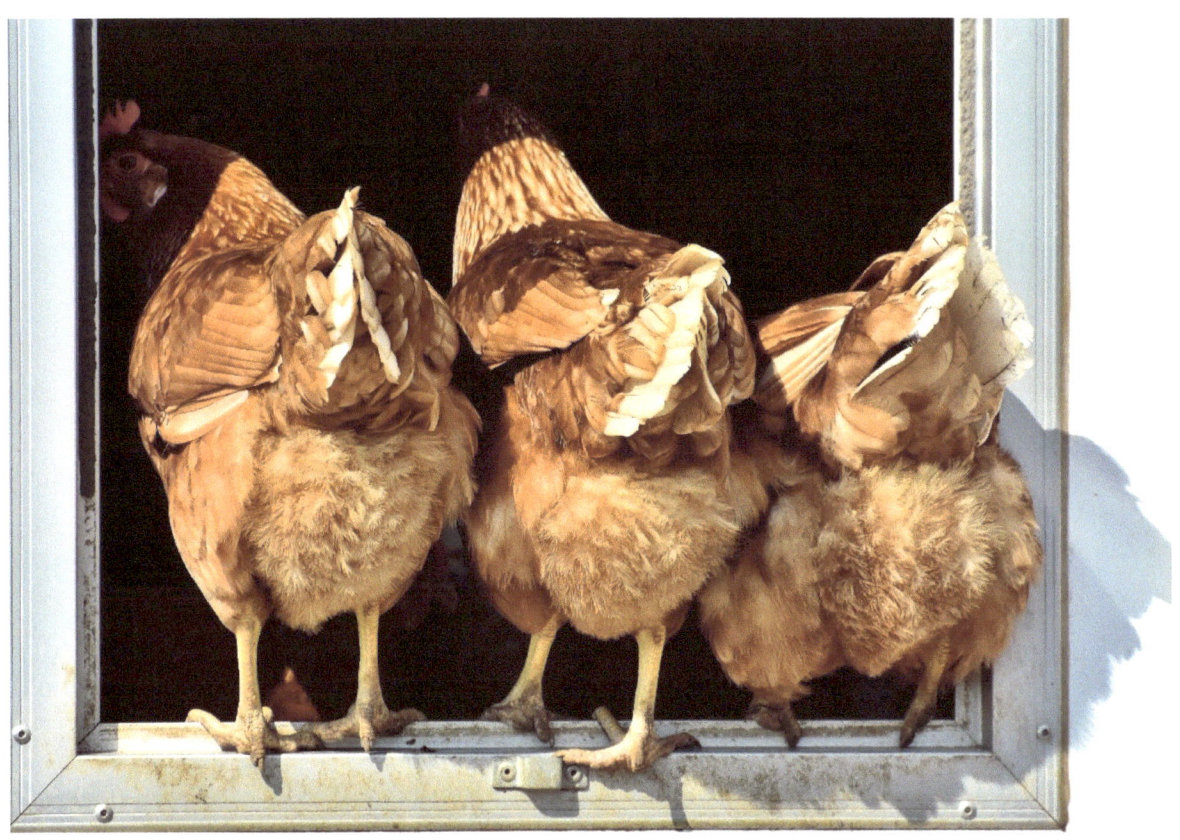

Grumbles from the Chuckwagon:
Lesson learned: if I don't make enough chicken soft tacos for the crew, my cowgirl's "outta soap" to wash my britches. Meanwhile, the cowboys are fresh as daisies. So, next time? You bet I'll cook extra if I want clean pants tomorrow!

Chrissy Hartmann

6.14 Stuffed Sausage Peppers

Serving Size: 1 Pepper
Servings: 6
Approximate Calories: 533

Ingredients:
- 6 bell peppers (green, red, or yellow)
- 3 Cups cooked wild rice
- 1 pound cooked spicy sausage
- 3 Tablespoon grapeseed oil
- 1 quart mushrooms, sliced
- 1 onion, sliced
- 3 tomatoes
- 8 ounces sharp cheddar cheese
- 1 can tomato juice

Instructions:
1. In mixing bowl, combine cooked wild rice, sliced mushrooms, diced tomatoes, only 4 ounces of shredded sharp cheddar cheese, and cooked sausage with 2 tablespoons of grapeseed oil. Mix well.
2. Remove tops and seeds from 6 bell peppers, rinse thoroughly.
3. Stuff peppers with mix to the brim.
4. Place peppers in a 9×13 glass pan.
5. Use a basting brush, coat the peppers with the remaining grapeseed oil.
6. Pour tomato juice in with peppers so they wade in a shallow pool of juice.
7. Bake for 45 minutes at 350°F.
8. Once done, sprinkle remaining shredded cheddar cheese over peppers, if desired.
9. Enjoy with a nice crusty bread.

Nutritional Values:
% Daily Value based on a 2000 calorie diet

Total Fat 26 g	33%
Saturated Fat 11.3 g	57%
Cholesterol 107 mg	36%
Sodium 613 mg	27%
Carbohydrates 49.2 g	18%
Dietary Fiber 5 g	18%
Total Sugars 8 g	
Protein 42.2 g	

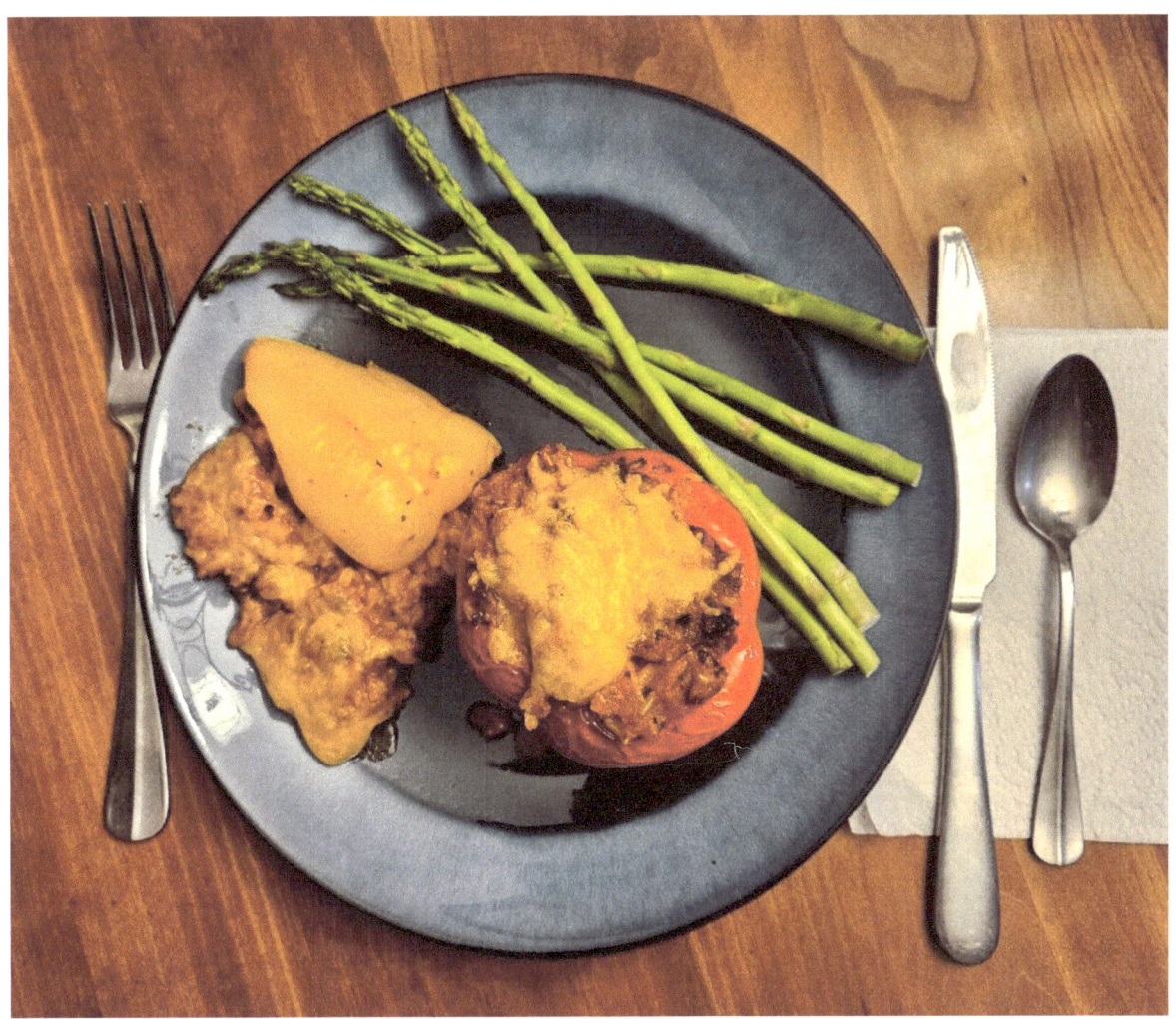

Grumbles from the Chuckwagon:
Had to wrestle this dish right outta the bosshand's grip at the hoedown. Fella figured he could hog it all. I told him, "You want the whole thing? Better learn to cook, because this ain't a one-man buffet!"

Chrissy Hartmann

6.15 Texas-Two Step Barbecue Chicken

Serving Size: 1 breast
Servings: 4
Approximate Calories: 228

Ingredients:
- 4 bone-in, skin-on chicken breasts
- Salt and pepper to season
- 1 cup barbecue sauce.
- 2 tablespoons Grapeseed oil

Instructions:
1. Preheat grill to medium-high heat.
2. In a bowl, whisk together all the BBQ sauce ingredients. Adjust seasoning to taste.
3. Lightly brush grapeseed oil over chicken, then season chicken with salt and pepper.
4. Brush the grill grates with grapeseed oil to prevent sticking. Place chicken on the grill, skin side down, and cook for 5-7 minutes until nicely seared.
5. Apply BBQ Sauce; flip the chicken, continue grilling, and brushing with BBQ sauce occasionally, until the internal temperature reaches 165°F and the chicken is cooked through.
6. Remove chicken from grill and let it rest for a few minutes. Serve the BBQ chicken with extra sauce on side.

Honey Barbecue Sauce

Ingredients:
- 1 cup ketchup
- 1/2 cup grapeseed oil
- 1/4 cup apple cider vinegar
- 1/4 cup honey
- 2 tablespoons Worcestershire sauce
- 1 tablespoon Dijon mustard
- 1 teaspoon smoked paprika
- 1 teaspoon garlic powder
- Salt and pepper to taste
- Optional: Liquid smoke to taste

Instructions:
1. Combine in medium-sized bowl.
2. Stir briskly until well blended. If sauce too thick, add 1 tablespoon of water for desired thickness.
3. Coat chicken on grill making sure to turn occasionally after reapplying.
4. Store in refrigerator when not in use.

Nutritional Value:
% daily value based on a 2000 calorie diet
Total Fat 7.5 g	10%
Saturated Fat 2 g	10%
Cholesterol 89 mg	30%
Sodium 366 mg	16%
Carbohydrates 9.1 g	3%
Dietary Fiber 0.2 g	1%
Total Sugars 6.5 g	
Protein 28.9 g	

Grumbles from the Chuckwagon:
When we say Texas-style, we mean plain and simple. So, Cowboys, when your cook's taking a much-needed rest, grilling up some chicken is as straightforward as it gets. Now, remember, the only hard part here is plucking those birds—no fancy frills on the prairie! So, fire up that grill, slather on the grapeseed oil-infused barbecue sauce, and enjoy a taste of the open range under the big old sky. And if you need more heat, add some cayenne pepper to the mix.

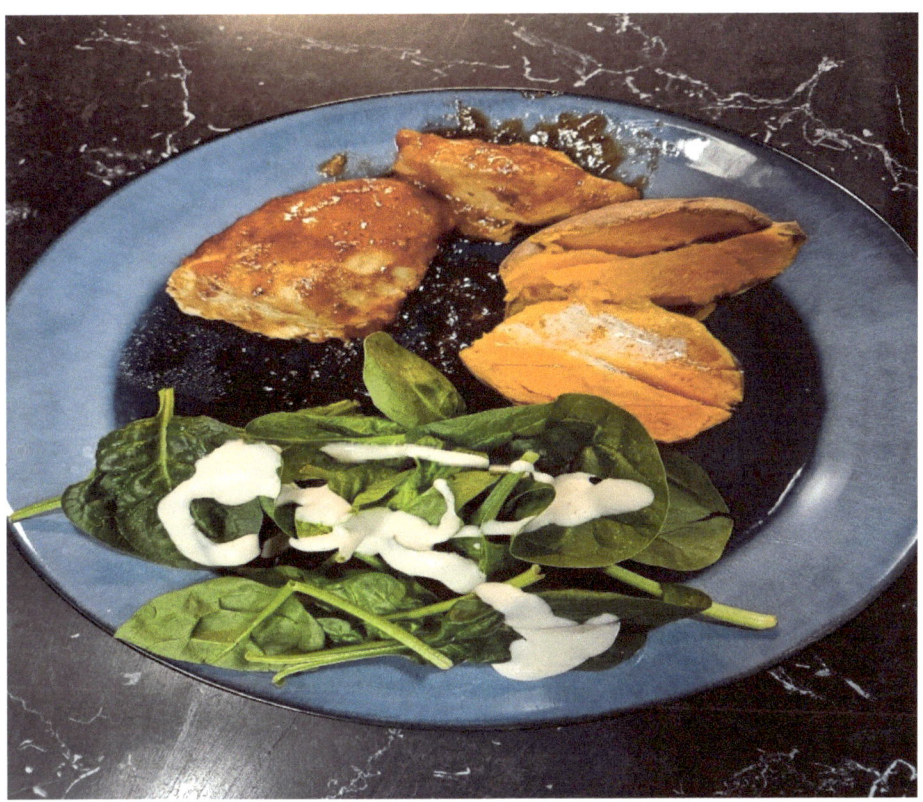

Chrissy Hartmann

6.16 Seared Salmon

Serving Size: 1 filet
Servings: 4
Approximate Calories: 63

Ingredients:
- 4 salmon fillets
- 2 tablespoons grapeseed oil
- Papa Fike's Original Seasoning to taste
- 1 lemon, sliced

Instructions:
1. Season salmon fillets with Papa Fike's Original Seasoning.
2. Heat grapeseed oil in a skillet over medium-high heat.
3. Place salmon fillets in the skillet, skin-side down.
4. Sear for a few minutes until skin is crispy and salmon is cooked through.
5. Garnish with lemon slices.

Nutritional Value:
% Daily Value based on a 2000 calorie diet

Total Fat 6.8 g	9%
Saturated Fat 0.7 g	3%
Cholesterol 0 mg	0%
Sodium 2 mg	0%
Carbohydrates 0.8 g	0%
Dietary Fiber 0.2 g	1%
Total Sugars 0.1 g	
Protein 0.2 g	

Grumbles from the Chuckwagon:
When the cowhands' bellies are grumbling like an old bear, what better to fix them to quiet down those hunger pains? That's right salmon. Not only does it put the kybosh on their hunger, but it's also a grand gesture toward the health of their tickers. And throwing a tossed salad or some brussel sprouts at my bears give me a hug to never forget.

6.17 Southwest Black Bean Burger

Serving Size: 1 burger
Servings: 5-6
Approximate Calories: 340

Ingredients:
- 2 15-ounce cans black beans, drained
- 1/2 cup corn
- 2/3 cups bread crumbs
- 2 teaspoon chipotle chili powder
- 1 egg
- 1 tablespoon grapeseed oil

Instructions:
1. In medium bowl, mash the black beans. Make sure to leave a few whole beans or pieces.
2. Mix into beans remaining ingredients except for grapeseed oil. Stir well.
3. Form mixture into bun-sized burger patties (about 5 ounces each).
4. Next, heat grapeseed oil in a large skillet over medium heat. Cook the patties for about 4-5 minutes on one side, then flip and cook for an additional 4-5 minutes. Prefer to bake, brush grapeseed oil both sides of burger patties. Bake at 375 °F for 10 minutes, flip halfway through.

Nutritional Value:
% Daily Value based on a 2000 calorie diet

Total Fat 8 g	12%
Saturated Fat 51 g	5%
Cholesterol 0 mg	0%
Sodium 540 mg	23%
Total Carbohydrates 27 g	13%
Dietary Fiber 9 g	36%
Total Sugars 3 g	
Protein 22 g	

Grumbles from the Chuckwagon:
Folks 'round the ranch had their boots all tangled up when for the first time, I dished out black bean burgers instead of the usual beefy delights. The cowboys were ready to brand me as a traitor, but hunger and curiosity got the better of them. With a skeptical glance, they took a bite. By the time the dust settled, those same cowboys who were ready to poke me with that hot iron were begging for seconds. Turns out them black bean burgers had more flavor than a summer sunrise, and I went from branded traitor to culinary hero quicker than a tumbleweed rolling in the wind. Lesson learned -- Never underestimate a cowboy's appetite for good grub, even if it isn't what they're used to.

Chrissy Hartmann

6.18 Cowboy Salad

Serving Size: 1 bowl
Servings: 4
Approximate Calories: 280

Ingredients:
- 1 head lettuce, chopped
- 1 can black beans
- 1 can chickpeas
- Optional: 1 avocado, diced
- 1 can corn
- 4 Roma tomatoes
- 1 red and orange pepper, diced
- 1 onion, diced
- 1 cup shredded cheddar cheese
- ½ cup homemade grapeseed oil mayo (See chapter 9)
- ½ cup grapeseed oil BBQ sauce (See chapter 9)
- 2 cups grilled chicken or steak
- Optional: ½ cup bacon bit crumbles

Instructions:
1. Wash and Chop lettuce and place into large bowl.
2. Dice green pepper, tomatoes, avocado, and onions, sprinkle in with lettuce.
3. Drain corn, chickpeas, and black beans, pour into bowl with other veggies.
4. Add grilled chicken or steak to veggies.
5. Make BBQ sauce and homemade mayo separately, then combine, mix well.
6. Pour mayo and BBQ sauce combination over veggies and toss
7. Sprinkle cheddar cheese and bacon bit crumbles over top salad
8. Chill in refrigerator until ready to serve

Nutrition Value:
% Daily Value based on a 2000 calorie diet

Total Fat 11.1 g	14%
Saturated Fat 4.3 g	21%
Cholesterol 39 mg	13%
Sodium 184 mg	8%
Carbohydrates 30.4 g	29%
Dietary Fiber 12.3 g	44%
Total Sugars 17.2 g	
Protein 25 g	

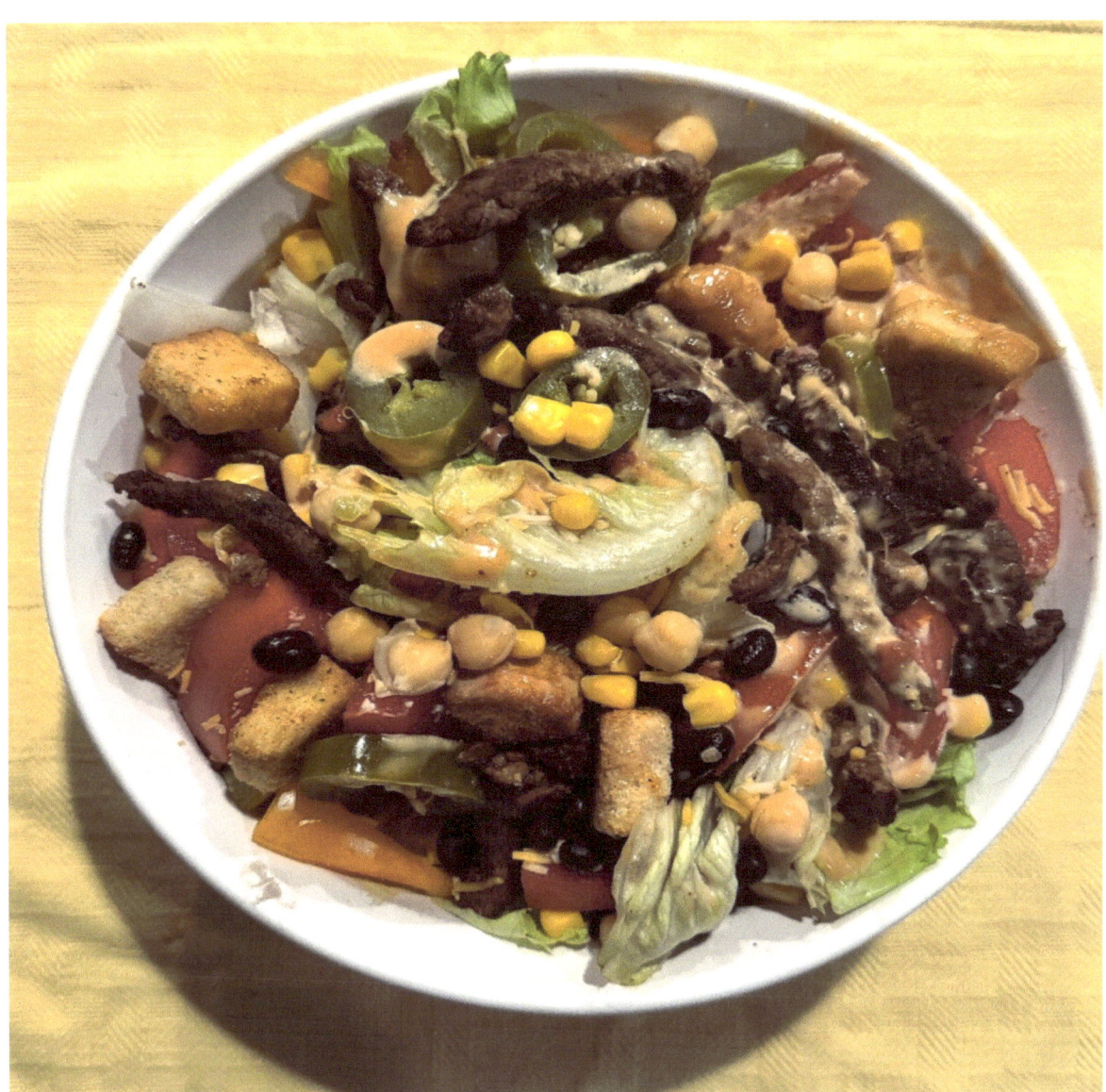

Grumbles from the Chuckwagon:
Well now, out on the trail, cowboys ain't too fond of salad—until I throw in my secret weapon: black beans and bacon crumbles. Once they smell that bacon, they're all in, like flies to honey. But if you're making something for the ladies, go without the beans. And between us? I ain't shy about enjoying a bowl myself, especially with my homemade dressing. So, when you need something green, just know the Grub Wrangler's got the best cowboy salad this side of the range.

Chrissy Hartmann

6.19 Calico Beans

Serving Size: 1
Servings: 6 – 8
Approximate Calories: 263

Ingredients:
- 1 tablespoon grapeseed oil
- 1 onion, diced
- 2 cloves garlic, minced
- 1 green bell pepper, diced
- 1 red bell pepper, diced
- 1 can (15 oz) kidney beans, drained and rinsed
- 1 can (15 oz) black beans, drained and rinsed
- 1 can (15 oz) pinto beans, drained and rinsed
- 1 can (15 oz) baked beans (with sauce)
- 1 can (15 oz) diced tomatoes
- 1/4 cup ketchup
- 2 tablespoons brown sugar
- 2 tablespoons cider vinegar
- 1 tablespoon Worcestershire sauce
- Salt and pepper to taste
- Optional: 1/2 cup cooked and crumbled bacon

Instructions:
1. Heat grapeseed oil in large skillet over medium heat. Add diced onion and cook until softened, about 5 minutes.
2. Add minced garlic, diced green and red bell peppers to skillet. Cook for another 3-4 minutes until peppers are tender.
3. In a large pot or Dutch oven, combine kidney beans, black beans, pinto beans, baked beans, diced tomatoes, ketchup, brown sugar, cider vinegar, Worcestershire sauce, and cooked onion-pepper mixture.
4. Bring mixture to a simmer over medium-low heat. Let it simmer uncovered for 30-40 minutes, stirring occasionally, until flavors are well blended, and beans are heated through.
5. Season with salt and pepper to taste.
6. If using bacon, stir in cooked and crumbled bacon at this point.
7. Serve hot. This dish can be enjoyed as a main course with taters or as a hearty side dish.

Nutrition Value:
% Daily Value based on a 2000 calorie diet

Total Fat 13.2 g	17.2 %
Saturated Fat 01.3 g	7 %
Cholesterol 0 mg	0%
Sodium 186 mg	8.3%
Carbohydrates 50.6 g	18%
Dietary Fiber 7 g	25%
Total Sugars 18.5 g	
Protein 10.3 g	

Grumbles from the Chuckwagon:
Well, let me tell ya, I nearly got left behind for forgetting the taters. Old Slim asked about them, and I said, "Ain't no taters today." You'd think I'd shot their prize bull from the way they looked at me. Calico Beans without taters? Might as well be watering down whiskey. Lesson learned—never forget a cowboy's taters for these here beans, or you're as good as gone!

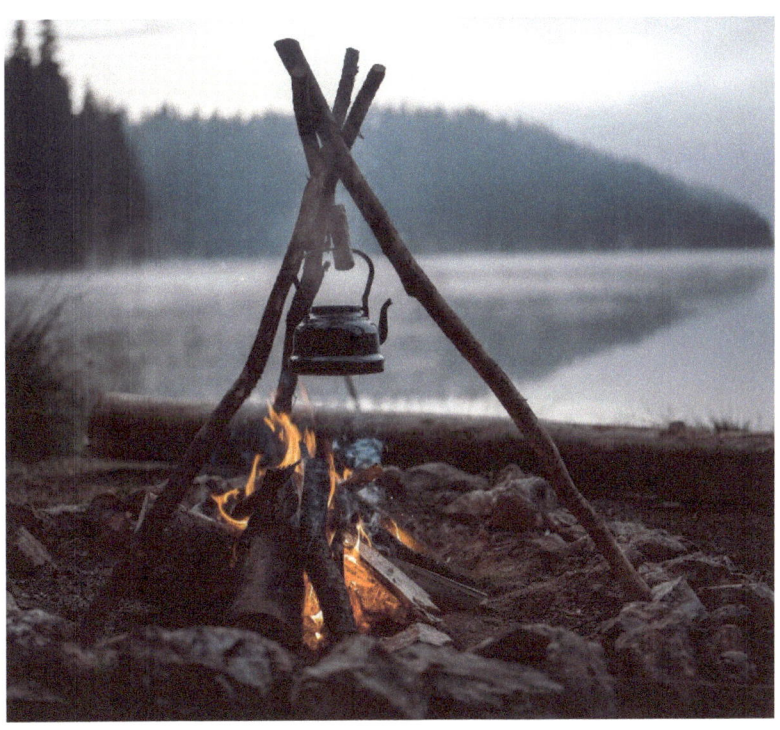

Chrissy Hartmann

The Grub Wrangler's Wisdom:

Chapter 7 Satisfying Sidekicks

In this chapter, we're talking sides that'll make your taste buds do a square dance. From crispy taters to cornbread with a golden crunch, each dish is infused with the goodness of grapeseed oil – the unsung hero that turns a simple side into a flavor stampede. And if them words don't explain it all, then how about this...

I had been wrangling up the fixings for our side dishes when I noticed something missing. Turns out, them key ingredients had done a vanishing act, and my search led me straight to a bunkhouse full of rodeo clowns. Seems the ranch agreed to host them for a spell while they geared up for the local rodeo.

Frustration boiled in my belly like a pot of cowboy coffee gone wrong. Them clowns were using my precious fixings as props for their circus antics, distracting horses, cattle, and who knows what else. Now, as we all know, side dishes are like the unsung heroes of a chuckwagon feast, especially when they're kissed by the magic of grapeseed oil. The thought of them being held hostage made me madder than a hornet in a rainstorm.

When the cowboys caught wind of the veggie hostage situation, well, they weren't too pleased. With a glint in their eyes, they took matters into their own hands, rustling them veggies away from them clowns faster than a cattle stampede.

In the end, the chuckwagon feast was saved, and them clowns learned a lesson about messing with a cowboy's grub, especially them fixings cooked up with the magic of grapeseed oil. Sometimes you gotta wrangle up your own veggies when the rodeo comes to town.

Remember now, sides are more than just supporting characters on your plate; they elevate the entire chuckwagon experience.

Here in these next pages, we'll showcase the versatility of grapeseed oil in crafting side dishes that not only tantalize your taste buds but also offer health benefits. Grapeseed oil's high smoke point ensures that these sides are cooked to perfection while retaining their nutritional value.

Remember grapeseed oil is the culinary partner that elevates these dishes, ensuring that your side dishes are just as satisfying and health conscious as the main grub. Enjoy these delectable side recipes that showcase the versatility of grapeseed oil in enhancing the chuckwagon experience.

So, grab your apron, and let's rustle up some sides that'll have your dinner guests talking about your cooking prowess from dusk 'til dawn.

Happy cooking, trailblazers!

Chrissy Hartmann

7.1 Yukon Golden Roasted Potatoes

Serving Size: 5 – 6 wedges
Servings: 8
Approximate Calories: 47

Ingredients:
- 2 pounds Yukon Golden potatoes (preferred)
- 3 tablespoons grapeseed oil
- 4 Garlic cloves, minced
- Fresh rosemary, 2 sprigs, leaves removed and chopped
- Fresh thyme, 2 sprigs, leaves removed
- 1 teaspoon salt
- 1/2 teaspoon black pepper

Instructions:
1. Preheat oven to 420°F.
2. Wash the potatoes thoroughly to remove any dirt or debris. Cut into bite size pieces.
3. In large bowl, combine the grapeseed oil, minced garlic, chopped rosemary, thyme leaves, salt, and black pepper. Mix well.
4. Add potato pieces to bowl and toss them gently to coat evenly with the grapeseed oil mixture.
5. Transfer potatoes to baking sheet. Spread out in a single layer.
6. Roast in oven for 50-60 minutes, make sure to flip over halfway through to brown both sides.
7. Remove from oven, let cool so the potatoes will crisp up.
8. Serve warm with main dish or with condiments as an appetizer.

Nutritional Value:
% Daily Value based on a 2000 calorie diet

Total Fat 5.1 g	7%
Saturated Fat 0.5 g	3%
Cholesterol 0 mg	0%
Sodium 291 mg	13%
Carbohydrates 0.4 g	0%
Dietary Fiber 0.2 g	1%
Total Sugars 0 g	
Protein 0.1 g	

Grumbles from the Chuckwagon:
Truly golden delights. These here taters are the simplest tasty side dish that everyone can make. They'll fill a cowboy's belly up. You can even add a little salsa to spice them up. And don't forget about serving them up with those calico beans! No matter what, no cowboy will go hungry with these little beauties.

7.2 Mediterranean Lemon Salad

Serving Size: 1 cup
Servings: 4
Approximate Calories: 170

Ingredients:
- Mixed greens
- 1 cup Lemon vinaigrette dressing (see chapter 9 for recipe)
- 1 cucumber, thinly sliced
- 4 Roma tomatoes, diced
- 1 jar pitted black olives, halved
- 1 can Chickpeas
- 1 red onion, sliced
- 4 ounces Feta cheese
- 1/4 cup almonds, sliced

Instructions:
1. Make lemon vinaigrette.
2. Dress salad crisper than autumn leaves and place it in large bowl, drizzle half the lemon vinaigrette over greens. Toss gently.
3. Add prepared tomatoes, cucumbers, black olives, chickpeas, and red onion. Toss together with remaining dressing.
4. Finish with Feta and almonds. Fluff gently.
5. Chill until ready to serve

Nutritional Value:
% Daily Value based on a 2000 calorie diet

Total Fat 9.6 g	12%
Saturated Fat 4.5 g	23%
Cholesterol 25 mg	8%
Sodium 331 mg	14%
Carbohydrates 16.1 g	6%
Dietary Fiber 4.1 g	15%
Total Sugars 8.7 g	
Protein 7.8 g	

Grumbles from the Chuckwagon:
Okay, she's a real beauty, right? Every once in a while, I like to switch things up. Yeh sure, the cowboys aren't crazy about it, but when dished out as a side, their plates always come up empty by meals end. Nice touch to add with salmon or chicken.

Chrissy Hartmann

7.3 Mushroom Onion Spinach Saute

Serving Size: 1 cup
Servings: 4
Approximate Calories: 76

Ingredients:
- 1 tablespoon grapeseed oil
- 1 large onion, sliced
- 1 quart baby Bella mushrooms, sliced
- 4 cups fresh spinach, chopped
- 2 cloves of garlic, minced
- 1 – 2 teaspoons balsamic vinegar
- Salt and pepper to taste

Instructions:
1. Preheat saute pan on medium heat with grapeseed oil.
2. Add onions and mushrooms, stirring for 5-10 minutes, until golden brown, adding garlic halfway through.
3. Add spinach and stir a minute or two, until spinach is just wilted.
4. Remove from heat and add balsamic vinegar, salt and pepper to taste.

Nutritional Values:
% Daily Value based on a 2000 calorie diet

Total Fat 3.7 g	5%
Saturated Fat 0.4 g	2%
Cholesterol 0 mg	0%
Sodium 30 mg	1%
Carbohydrates 9.6 g	3%
Dietary Fiber 2.7 g	10%
Total Sugars 3.5 g	
Protein 3 g	

Grumbles from the Chuckwagon:
Always thought the cowboys on the ranch were picky eaters. This side changed my mind. With the flavor of the onions, mushrooms, and spinach getting a little kick from the balsamic vinegar, it's hard to keep them from coming back for seconds. Very popular side when grilling beef, pork, or salmon. And for those who want a little more kick, try adding some of Papa Fike's Original Seasoning to it. Boy howdy, now that's a fabulous saute!

7.4 Green Bean Roundup with Bacon

Serving Size: 1 cup
Servings: 6
Approximate Calories: 128

Ingredients:
- 1 1/2 lb. fresh green beans, blanched and chilled
- salt, to taste
- 4 tablespoons grapeseed oil
- 3 cloves garlic, chopped
- Ground black pepper, to taste
- 4 strips cooked bacon, crumbled (optional)

Instructions:
1. Trim stem end from the green beans.
2. Heat pot of water over high heat until boiling. Season generously with salt.
3. Add green beans, cook for 3 to 5 minutes, until tender, yet still crisp. Drain and rinse under cold water to cool.
4. Return pot to medium heat. Add grapeseed oil and garlic. Cook for 1 minute, until fragrant.
5. Add beans and bacon crumbles to pot and stir gently to combine.
6. Add salt and pepper to taste.
7. Serve immediately.

Nutritional Value:
% Daily Value based on a 2000 calorie diet

Total Fat 9.3 g	12%
Saturated Fat 0.9 g	5%
Cholesterol 0 mg	0%
Sodium 397 mg	17%
Carbohydrates 11 g	4%
Dietary Fiber 5.2 g	19%
Total Sugars 2.1 g	
Protein 2.8 g	

Grumbles from the Chuckwagon:
Garlic green beans with bacon sprinkled with fresh ground black pepper – they're the Texas cowboy of your plate – robust, a little spicy, and full of character. The garlic adds grit, the pepper brings the kick, creating a culinary rodeo that mirrors the bold Texan cowboys.

Chrissy Hartmann

7.5 Campfire Roasted Asparagus

Serving Size: 4 Stalks
Servings: 6
Approximate Calories: 85

Ingredients:
- 2 pounds fresh asparagus, trimmed
- 1/4 cup grapeseed oil
- 4 teaspoons grated lemon zest
- 2 garlic cloves, minced
- 1/2 teaspoon salt
- 1/2 teaspoon pepper
- Toasted pine nuts

Instructions:
1. Heat skillet on medium high heat with grapeseed oil
2. Add minced garlic and stir.
3. Place trimmed and washed asparagus in skillet, rotate every few minutes.
4. Sprinkle remaining ingredients over asparagus. Rotate to coat.
5. Fry until crisp-tender, 12 -15 minutes.
6. Serve with toasted pine nuts.

Nutritional Values:
% Daily Value based on a 2000 calorie diet

Total Fat 7.1 g	9%
Saturated Fat 0.7 g	4%
Cholesterol 0 mg	0%
Sodium 150 mg	7%
Carbohydrates 4.7 g	2%
Dietary Fiber 2.5 g	9%
Total Sugars 2.2 g	
Protein 2.6 g	

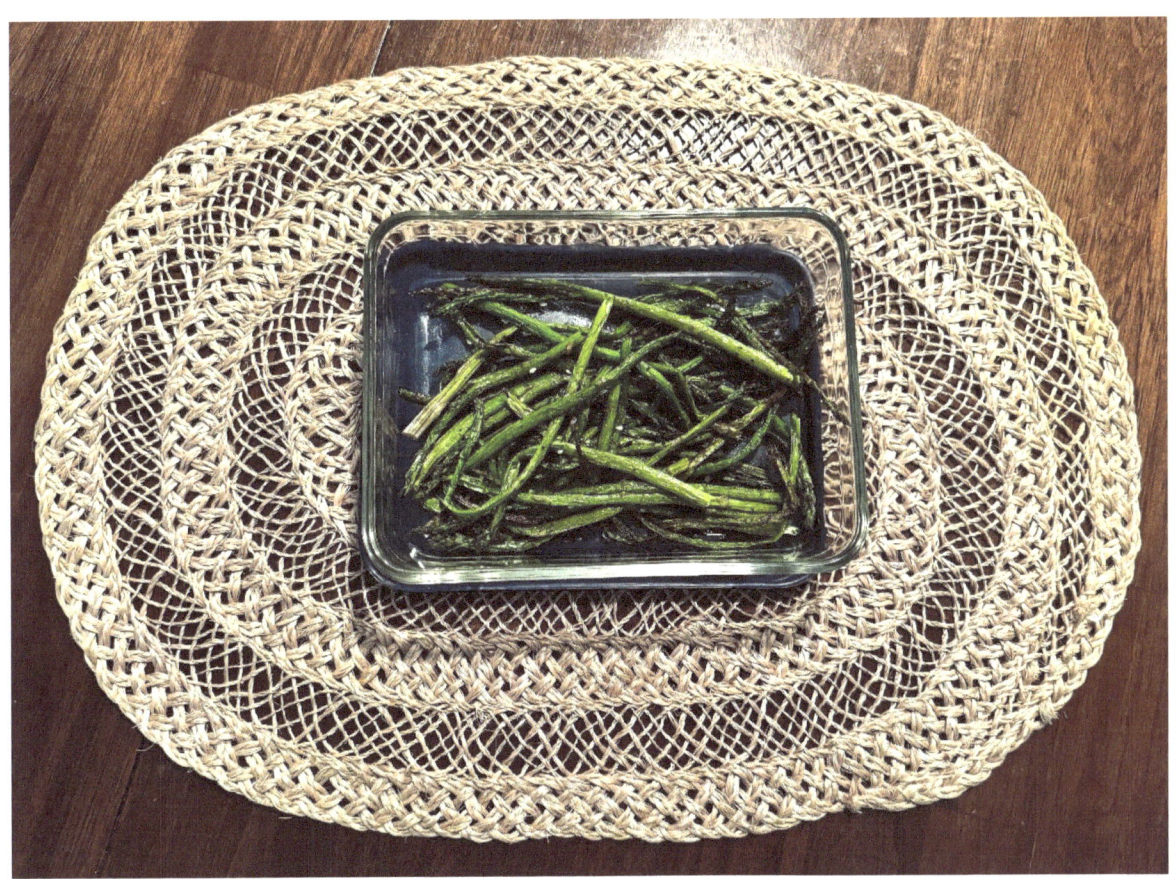

Grumbles from the Chuckwagon:
These tender, but flavorful spears that are nicely pan fried over the campfire have many nutrients, but low on the calories. And nobody wants an overweight cowboy, right? And you know those good-looking cowboys? How do you think they keep their good looks? Yep, asparagus. Loaded with lots of antioxidants that help keep you looking young while out in the hot sun. Now don't take that wrong, I'm not looking, but my cowgirl sure likes to keep an eye on those fellas. She doesn't want the cougars chasing them.

Chrissy Hartmann

7.6 Balsamic Glazed Carrots

Serving Size: 1 cup
Servings: 4
Approximate Calories: 120

Ingredients:
- 1 pound baby carrots, cleaned and trimmed
- 2 tablespoons grapeseed oil
- 3 tablespoons balsamic glaze
- 1 tablespoon honey
- 1 teaspoon Dijon mustard
- Salt and black pepper to taste
- Fresh parsley, chopped (for garnish, optional)

Instructions:
1. Preheat oven to 400°F.
2. In small bowl, toss the baby carrots with grapeseed oil, salt, and pepper until evenly coated.
3. Spread carrots on baking sheet in single layer. Roast in preheated oven for 20-25 minutes or until carrots are tender and slightly caramelized.
4. In small saucepan, combine balsamic glaze, honey, and Dijon mustard. Cook over medium heat, stirring constantly until mixture thickens slightly (about 3-5 minutes).
5. Once carrots are done, transfer to a serving dish. Pour balsamic glaze mixture over roasted carrots, ensuring they are well coated.
6. Garnish and if desired, sprinkle chopped fresh parsley over glazed carrots for a burst of freshness. Serve immediately.

Nutritional Values:
% daily value based on a 2000 calorie diet

Total Fat 7 g	10%
Saturated Fat 1 g	5%
Trans Fat 0 g	0%
Cholesterol 0 mg	0%
Sodium 180 mg	8%
Carbohydrates 15 g	15%
Dietary Fiber: 3 g	12%
Sugars: 9 g	18%
Protein 1 g	2%

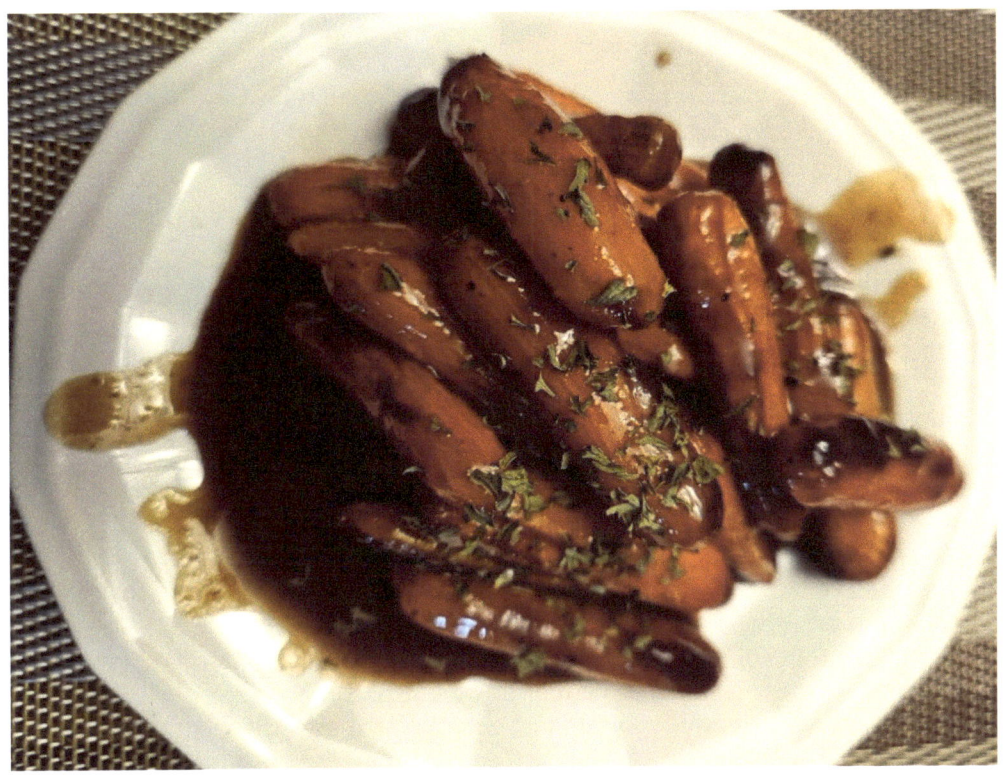

Grumbles from the Chuckwagon:
This is no bunny ranch, but even the jack rabbits will be wanting these for dinner. Not only good for the eyes, but a heart healthy side that bursts with flavor and lots of nutrients. No cowboy should do without.

Chrissy Hartmann

7.7 Lonestar Tater Salad

Serving Size: 1/2 cup
Servings: 8
Approximate Calories: 267

Ingredients:
- 1 - 2 pounds red potatoes, boiled and diced
- 4 eggs boiled and diced
- 1/2 cup celery, finely chopped
- 1/4 cup red onion, finely chopped
- 1 cup Homemade Mayo (see chapter 9)
- 1 tablespoons Dijon mustard
- black pepper to taste

Instructions:
1. In large pan, boil red potatoes and eggs 20-30 minutes, until potatoes are fork tender. Allow them to cool and then dice.
2. In large bowl, combine diced potatoes, eggs, celery, and red onion.
3. Stir in Homemade Mayo and black pepper until gently combined.
4. Chill potato salad in refrigerator for at least 1 hour. Garnish with fresh dill before serving.

Nutritional Value:
% daily value based on a 2000 calorie diet

Total Fat 23.3 g	30%
Saturated Fat 4 g	20%
Cholesterol 103 mg	34%
Sodium 369 mg	16%
Carbohydrates 11.4 g	4%
Dietary Fiber 4.1 g	15%
Total Sugars 0.8 g	
Protein 5.4 g	

Grumbles from the Chuckwagon:
This creamy tater Salad, dressed in a grapeseed oil based mayo and pepper is a crowd-pleaser. A perfect balance of heat and creaminess, it's a must-have at any chuckwagon gathering. A Dijon vinaigrette is also a good choice if some of your cowboys don't partake in mayo-based dishes.

7.8 Lemon Broccoli

Serving Size: 1/2 cup
Servings: 4
Approximate calories: 83

Ingredients:
- 1 lb broccoli florets
- 2 garlic cloves, minced
- 2 tablespoons grapeseed oil
- Zest and juice of 1 lemon
- Salt and black pepper to taste

Instructions:
1. Steam broccoli until just tender, about 3-4 minutes. Drain.
2. In pan, heat grapeseed oil. Add minced garlic and sauté until fragrant.
3. Toss blanched broccoli into the pan. Stir in lemon zest and juice.
4. Season with salt and black pepper. Stir well and serve.

Nutritional Values:
% daily value Based on a 2000 calorie diet

Total Fat 0.3 g	0%
Saturated Fat 0 g	0%
Cholesterol 0 mg	0%
Sodium 17 mg	1%
Carbohydrates 18.2 g	7%
Dietary Fiber 1.7 g	6%
Total Sugars 0.9 g	
Protein 3.9 g	

Grumbles from the Chuckwagon:
Not fond of a greenhorn practicing his lasso tosses. Not aware that he had an audience, he did a fancy twist of his wrist and sent the rope whirling. Positive the target had to be those old longhorns over the fireplace, but as they came nowhere catching hold of them, I realized too late it had been the pile of broccoli I worked on. I saw the orneriness spark in that young cowboy's eyes, and he flicked his wrist again and snagged a bunch of the greens. Amused by his catch, he gave a triumphant tug sending a bunch of them through the air. Once he reclaimed the airborne broccoli, he declared it a new cowboy trick. And years later, there's still Nothing like roping in those broccoli florets, except I do it with a lemon garlic lasso.

Chrissy Hartmann

7.9 Spicy Sweet Taters

Serving Size: 4 wedges
Servings: 8
Approximate Calories: 165

Ingredients:
- 2 large, sweet potatoes cut into wedges
- 2 tablespoons grapeseed oil
- 1 teaspoon chili powder
- 1/2 teaspoon smoked paprika
- 1/2 teaspoon cumin
- Salt to taste

Instructions:
1. Preheat oven to 400°F.
2. Cut sweet taters into wedges.
3. In medium bowl, toss sweet tater wedges with grapeseed oil, chili powder, smoked paprika, cumin, and salt until well coated.
4. Spread wedges on baking sheet. Bake for 45-60 minutes or until crispy.
5. Transfer to serving dish and serve hot.

Nutritional Values:
% daily value based on a 2000 calorie diet

Total Fat 7 g	12%
Saturated Fat 0.5 g	3%
Trans Fat 0 g	0%
Cholesterol 0 mg	0%
Sodium 150 mg	6%
Total Carbohydrates 24 g	12%
Dietary Fiber: 4 g	16%
Sugars: 6 g	12%
Protein 2 g	4%

Grumbles from the Chuckwagon:
No real grumbles today, but a certain cowgirl showed up one day at the back of my chuckwagon begging I make these here sweet ones with a little more fixings to them. Now she said if I made them, she'd return the favor. So, after getting all the ingredients I made them. Now boy howdy! These Spicy Sweet Taters , doused in grapeseed oil, are a flavor explosion on the taste buds. A fiery kick for those bronco-busting cowboys and gals who don't have enough heat in their life and need a little more than regular taters. And if you're wondering, did my cowgirl grant me a favor? Well, I don't kiss and tell, so, we'll have to leave it at that.

7.10 Pony Up Pasta Salad

Serving Size: 1 cup
Servings: 4
Approximate Calories: 250

Ingredients:
- 1 pound tri-color pasta, cooked al dente
- 1 cup cherry tomatoes, halved
- 1 cup bell pepper, sliced
- 1/4 cup banana pepper rings
- 1/2 cup olives, sliced
- 1 cup cubed mozzarella
- 1/2 cup grapeseed oil
- 1/2 cup balsamic vinegar
- Salt and black pepper to taste
- Optional: 1/3 cup parsley or basil

Instructions:
1. Cook pasta according to package instructions. Drain and let it cool.
2. In large bowl, combine pasta, cherry tomatoes, bell pepper, banana peppers, olives, mozzarella, and chopped basil.
3. In small bowl, whisk together grapeseed oil, balsamic vinegar, salt, and black pepper.
4. Pour dressing over pasta mixture, toss until evenly coated.
5. Chill in refrigerator for at least 30 minutes before serving. Serve cold.

Nutritional Value:
% daily value based on a 2000 calorie diet

Total Fat 10 g	15%
- Saturated Fat 4 g	20%
- Trans Fat 0 g	0%
- Cholesterol 15 mg	5%
- Sodium 150 mg	6%
- Total Carbohydrates 30 g	10%
- Dietary Fiber: 6 g	20%
- Sugars: 4 g	8%
- Protein 10 g	20%

Grumbles from the Chuckwagon:
This lite pasta salad hasn't crossed one set of cowboy lips that didn't like it. In fact, it's requested quite often. With no heavy oils or mayo, it makes for a quick salad to rustle up for those days the cowboys need to pony up and keep moving the herd.

Chrissy Hartmann

7.11 Buckshot Brussel Sprouts

Serving Size: 1 cup
Servings: 4
Approximate Calories: 80

Ingredients:
- 1 pound Brussels sprouts, trimmed and quartered
- 1 tablespoon grapeseed oil
- 1/4 cup maple syrup
- Salt and black pepper to taste
- 1/4 cup chopped walnuts

Instructions:
1. Preheat oven to 400°F.
2. Cut stem off each brussel sprout and quarter.
3. In bowl, toss Brussel sprouts with grapeseed oil, maple syrup, salt, black pepper, and walnuts until well coated.
4. Spread Brussel sprouts on baking sheet. Roast for 25-30 minutes or until golden and crispy on edges.
5. Transfer to serving dish and serve immediately.

Nutritional Values:
% daily value based on a 2000 calorie diet

Total Fat 39.9 g	51%
Saturated Fat 3.3 g	16%
Trans Fat 0 g	0%
Cholesterol 0 mg	0%
Sodium 7 mg	0%
Total Carbohydrates 8.9 g	3%
Dietary Fiber: 2.6 g	9%
Total Sugars: 4.5 g	7%
Protein 6.9 g	9%

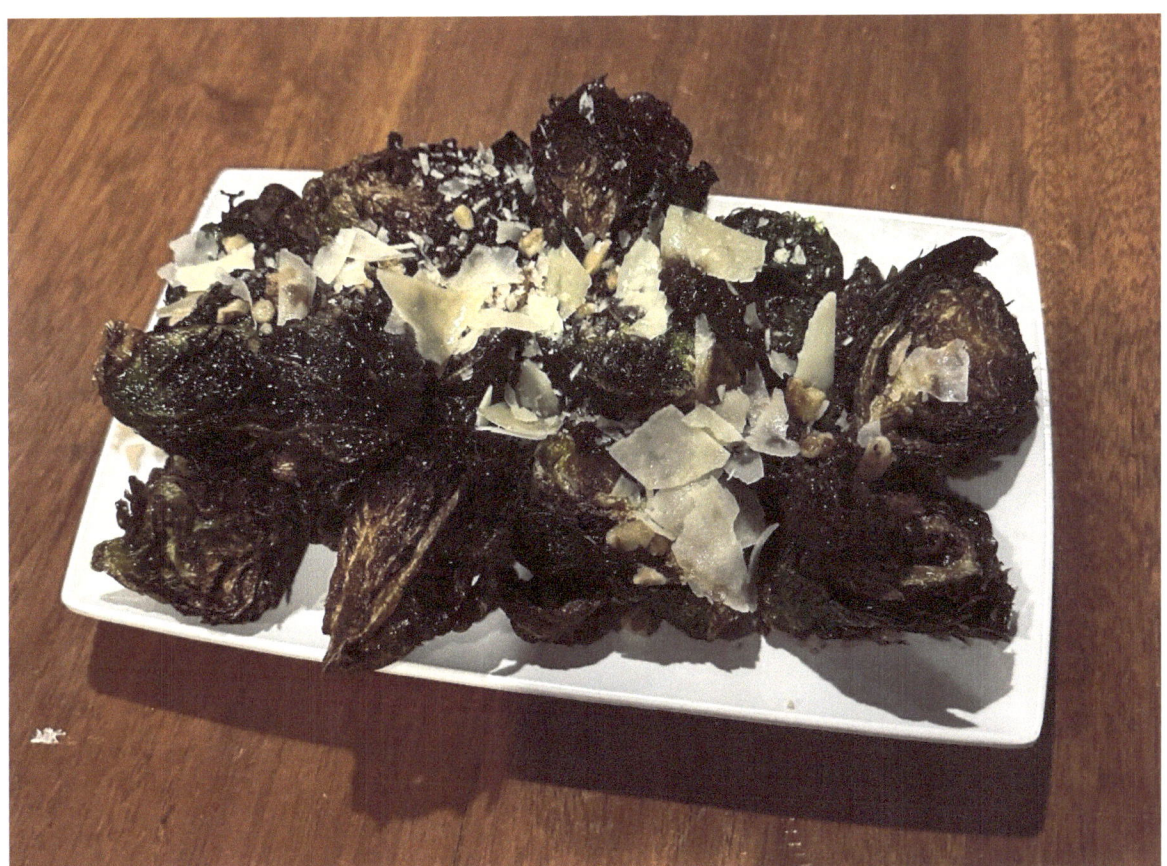

Grumbles from the Chuckwagon:
These are a game changer! After a long hard day branding cattle or riding the trails, the cowboys find it enjoyable to sit down at sunset and enjoy these delicious beauties with a nice steak or side of pork. Their sweet nutty flavor makes the day's work fade away. And best of all, you can change up the sauce for them. Just check out the different sauces in chapter 9. And just between us, adding bacon bits to these tasty bites will make you the favorite around the chuckwagon.

Chrissy Hartmann

7.12 Crispy Chipotle Kale Chips

Serving Size: 1/2 cup
Servings: 8
Approximate Calories: 267

Ingredients:
1-2 bunches of kale, stems removed, and leaves torn into bite-sized pieces
- 2 tablespoons grapeseed oil
- 1/2 teaspoon garlic powder
- 2 teaspoons chipotle
- Salt to taste

Instructions:
1. Preheat oven to 350°F.
2. In large bowl, massage kale leaves with grapeseed oil, garlic powder, chipotle, and salt until well coated.
3. Spread kale leaves in single layer on baking sheet. Bake for 12-15 minutes or until edges are crispy.
4. Allow kale chips to cool before serving. Enjoy as crunchy and healthy snack.

Nutritional Values:
% daily value based on a 2000 calorie diet

Total Fat 25.9 g	33%
Saturated Fat 2.5 g	13%
Cholesterol 0 mg	0%
Sodium 9 mg	0%
Carbohydrates 9.3 g	3%
Dietary Fiber 3.2 g	11%
Total Sugars 2.2 g	
Protein 2.3 g	

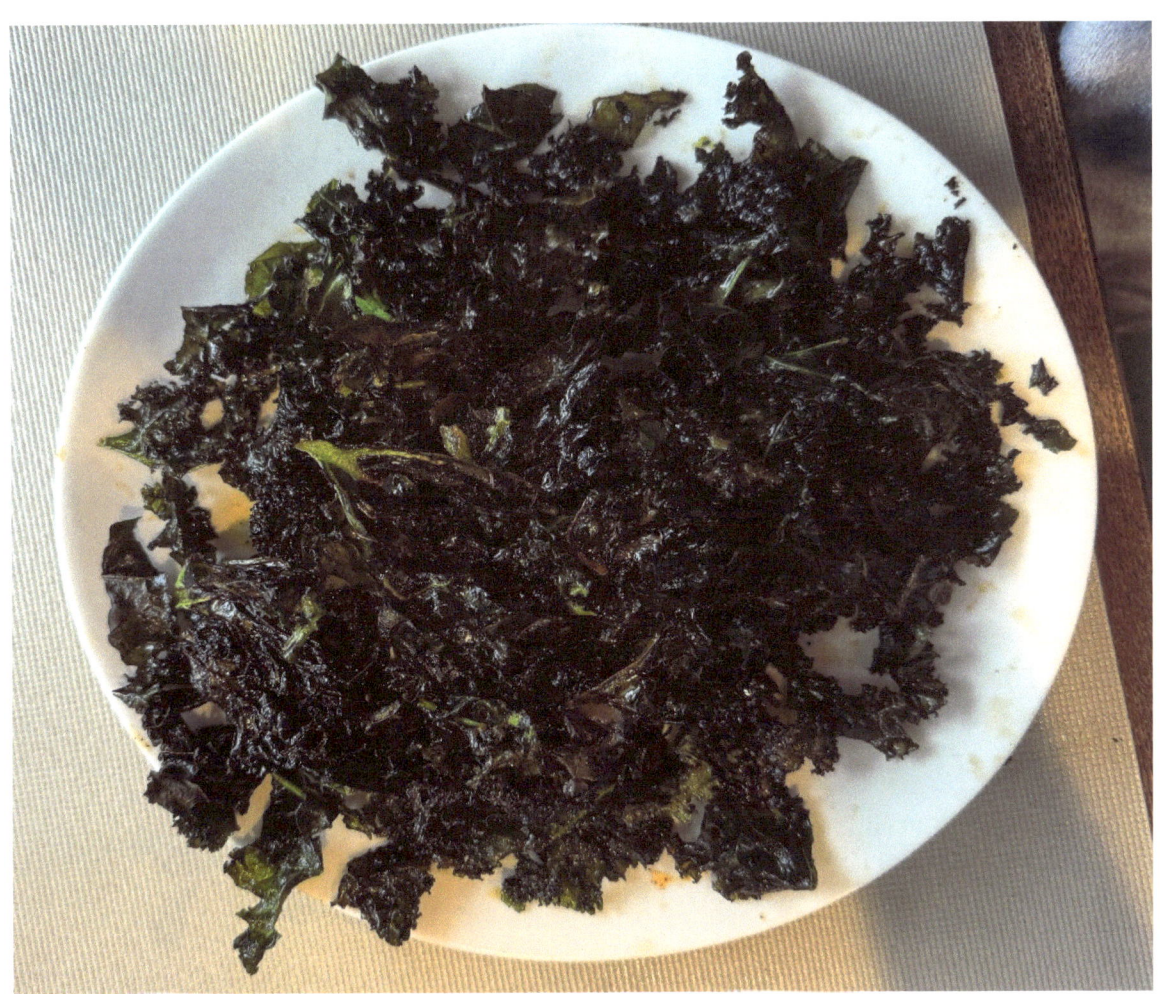

Grumbles from the Chuckwagon:

There's no telling how many of these I've made. Maybe as many as the stars fill the vast Texas sky. No matter what, they too seem to disappear before the night's over. These Crispy Chipotle Kale Chips, crisped up with a touch of grapeseed oil, are like bites of prairie stardust. A fabulous side for tuna melts or your catfish dinner. And a guilt-free snack that's sure to keep you munching on the trail.

Chrissy Hartmann

7.13 Chuckwagon Cornbread

Serving Size 1 square
Servings: 8
Approximate Calories: 208

Ingredients:
- 1 cup cornmeal
- 1 cup all-purpose flour
- 1 tablespoon baking powder
- 1/2 teaspoon salt
- 1 cup buttermilk
- 1/2 cup grapeseed oil
- 2 large eggs
- 1/4 cup honey

Instructions:
1. Preheat oven to 400°F and grease baking pan or cast-iron skillet with grapeseed oil.
2. In large bowl, sift together to resemble desert sand cornmeal, flour, baking powder, and salt.
3. In separate bowl, combine buttermilk, grapeseed oil, eggs, and honey, mix well.
4. Combine wet and dry ingredients and stir until just mixed.
5. Pour batter into prepared pan and smooth top.
6. Bake for 20-25 minutes Letting dough rise like morning sun, until toothpick inserted into center comes out clean.
7. Cool in pan for few minutes, then transfer to wire rack to cool completely.
8. Slice and serve with favorite spread.

Nutritional Value:
% daily value based on a 2000 calorie diet
Total Fat 9.5 g 12%
Saturated Fat 1.5 g 8%
Cholesterol 94 mg 31%
Sodium 2487 mg 108%
Carbohydrates 28.4 g 10%
Dietary Fiber: 1.5 g 6%
Sugars: 3.5 g
Protein 5.9 g

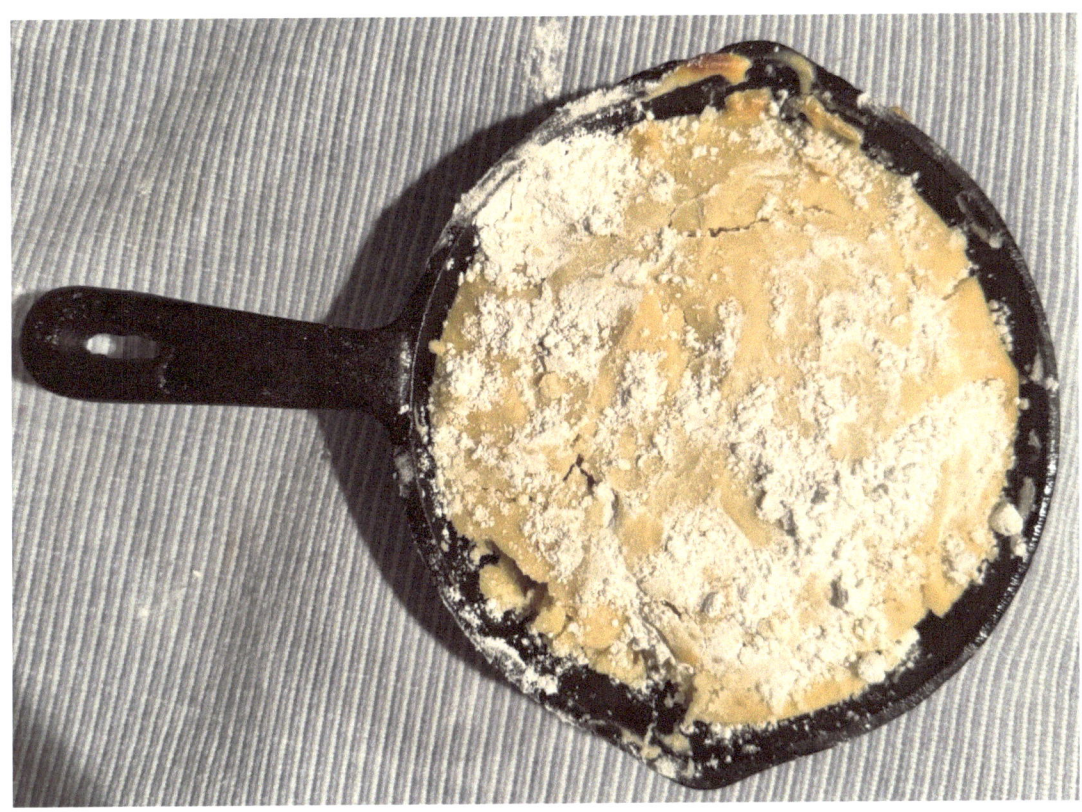

Grumbles from the Chuckwagon:
Nothing like making the cowboys feel appreciated. After all, why not. They do all the fence mending, branding, and cattle rustling when there's time. And with a day out on the range with lots of chores I've found that my cowboys love the simple things in life just a bit more. And what fills their hearts with sweetness and love? Yep, that's right my cornbread. They adore the hearty simplicity of this cornbread. The grapeseed oil adds a touch of richness without overpowering the rugged flavors of the trail. It's an easy fix after a long day in the saddle—just mix, bake to the color of a harvest moon and savor the taste of home on the range.

Chrissy Hartmann

7.13 Texas Hash

Serving Size: 1 cup
Servings: 6
Approximate Calories: 312

Ingredients:
- 1 pound of ground beef or turkey
- 1-2 tablespoons grapeseed oil
- 1 cup uncooked rice.
- 1 teaspoon chili powder
- 1 onion chopped
- 1 green bell pepper, diced.
- 1 can of corn
- 1 can of tomato sauce
- 1 cup of black beans
- 1/2 cup shredded cheddar cheese

Instructions:
1. Cook rice, set on side.
2. Using grapeseed oil on medium heat, cook meat, green pepper, onion, and chili powder until meat is browned.
3. Add corn, black beans, and tomato sauce, mix well.
4. Add cooked rice while stirring until the rice and beans are well blended in.
5. Turn heat to low, add cheddar cheese and stir until melted.
6. Serve warm

Nutritional Value:
% daily value based on a 2000 calorie diet

Total Fat 23.8 g	31%
Saturated Fat 4.3 g	21%
Cholesterol 21 mg	7%
Sodium 326 mg	14%
Carbohydrates 41.7 g	15%
Dietary Fiber 10 g	36%
Total Sugars 4.9 g	
Protein 15.2 g	

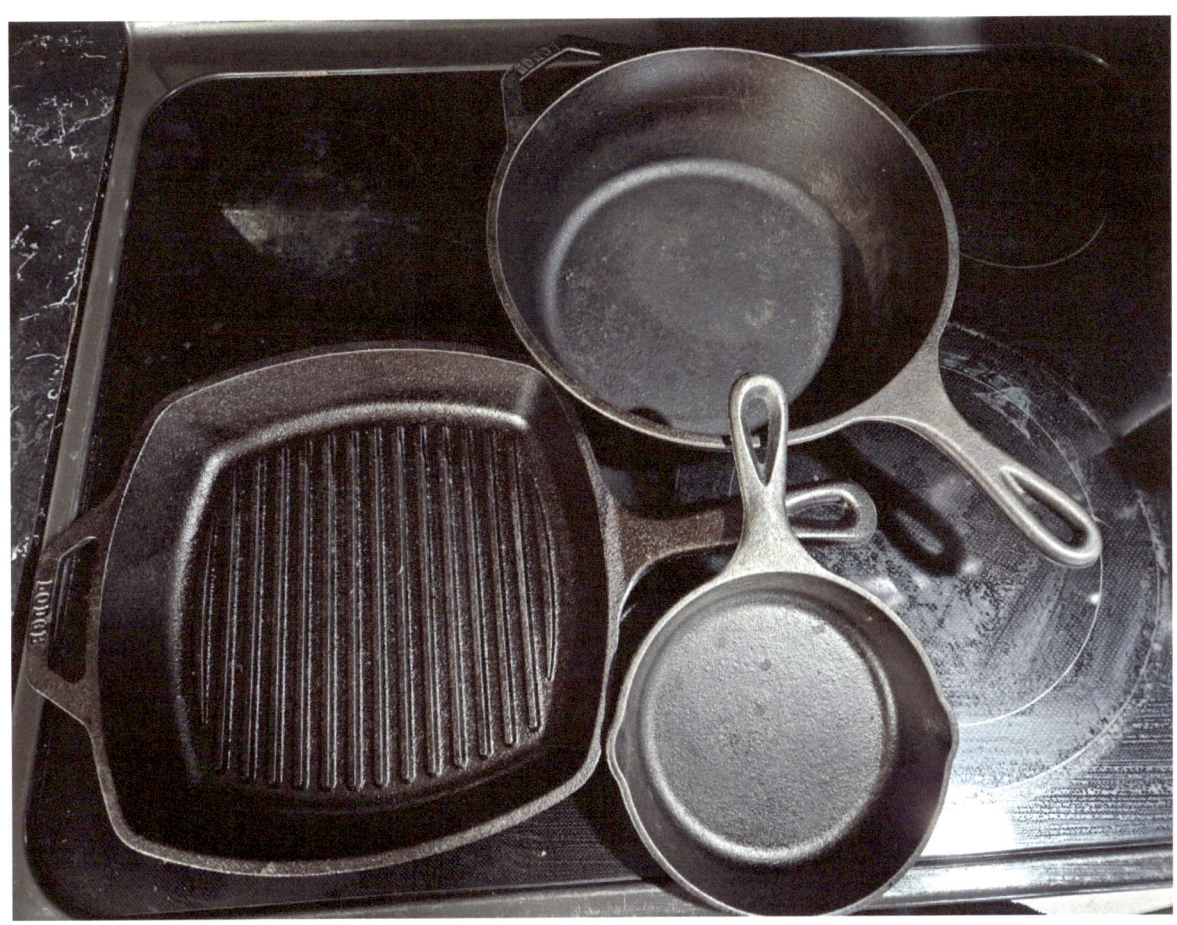

Grumbles from the Chuckwagon:
Sometimes this here dish serves as a side and sometimes as a main dish, it depends if we're out on the range or back at the ranch. The cowhands love it though. Seems like each time it's made they want something else thrown in. Mushrooms? Jalapenos? hey, whatever's put in next it only makes these boys here cowboy strong. So, cowboy up, cause the eating is good!

Chrissy Hartmann

The Grub Wrangler's Wisdom:

Chapter 8 Delicious Desserts

Grab your hat, partner! Welcome to "Delicious Desserts," where the sweet trail meets satisfaction. In this chapter, we're wrangling up some mighty fine treats with the secret weapon of the west– grapeseed oil. Just like the time I lassoed a blue ribbon in the community baking contest for my Texas sheet cake . Yup, that's correct. A blue ribbon.

Well, partner, let me spin that yarn a bit more. There I was, knee-deep in flour and determination, mixing up a batch of brownies that could make a coyote howl with delight. Now, the secret weapon? Grapeseed oil. It added a touch of sophistication to the richness, making those brownies the talk of the town. Fast forward to the community baking contest – judges were grinning like Cheshire cats after one bite, and before I knew it, I had that coveted blue ribbon in hand.

Now, about grapeseed oil – it's the unsung hero of the range. With a high smoke point and mild flavor, it lets the other ingredients shine without overpowering. Plus, it's packing antioxidants, making it a healthier choice for wranglers watching their waistlines… But only if they're watching those portion sizes too.

So, in the world of desserts, grapeseed oil ain't just a sidekick; it's the hero of the saloon, settling taste buds and winning ribbons one dessert at a time. Desserts are the sweet ending of a meal. And grapeseed oil brings a rich, delicate flavor that'll have folks hollering for seconds. So, grab your apron, dust off your cowboy hat, and let's rustle up some dessert magic!

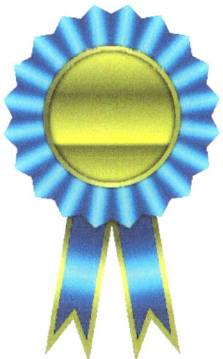

Chrissy Hartmann

8.1 Iowa Dusty Delights

Serving Size: 1 brownie
Servings: 12
Approximate Calories: 231

Ingredients:
- 1 cup dark chocolate chips
- 1/2 cup grapeseed oil
- 1 cup granulated sugar
- 3 large eggs
- 1 teaspoon pure vanilla extract
- 1/2 cup all-purpose flour
- 1/4 cup unsweetened cocoa powder
- 1/4 teaspoon salt
- powdered sugar to dust

Instructions:
1. Preheat oven to 350°F. Grease or line baking pan.
2. Melt dark chocolate chips with grapeseed oil over a double boiler or in microwave. Stir until smooth.
3. In separate bowl, whisk together sugar, eggs, and vanilla extract. Add melted chocolate mixture and mix well.
4. Sift to resemble desert sand flour, cocoa powder, and salt. Fold real gentle like a graceful dance partner until just combined.
5. Pour batter into prepared pan and spread it evenly. Bake for 25-30 minutes or until a toothpick inserted in center, comes out clean.
6. Allow brownies to cool completely in the pan on a wire rack.
7. Dust with powdered sugar and cut to serve.

Nutritional Value:
% Daily Value based on a 2000 calorie diet

Total Fat 13.3 g	17%
Saturated Fat 3.1 g	15%
Cholesterol 47 mg	16%
Sodium 68 mg	3%
Carbohydrates 28.4 g	10%
Dietary Fiber 0.7 g	3%
Total Sugars 22.2 g	
Protein 3.1 g	

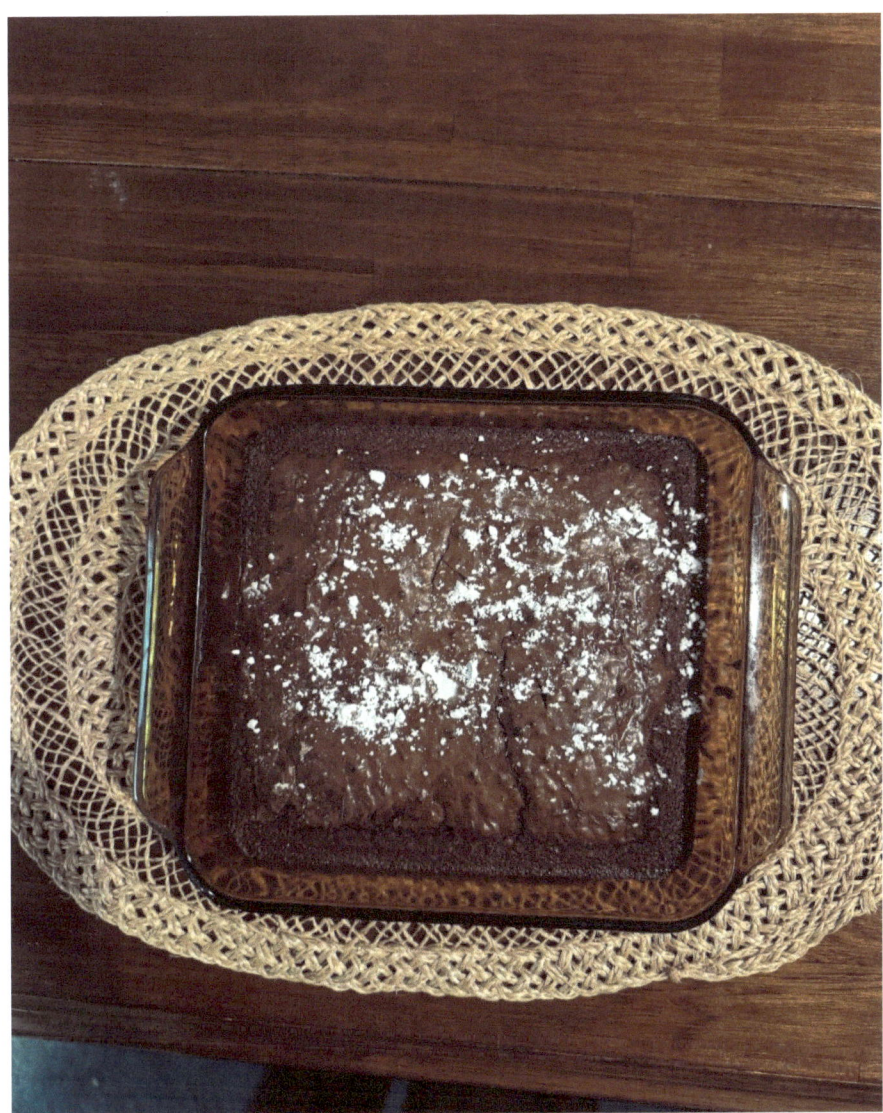

Grumbles from the Chuckwagon:
Typically, the disappearance of brownies is met with little fuss, but when Sweet Toothed Bandits destroyed my baking pan during their hasty departure, tolerance reached its limit. Vowing never to make those delights again, my threat was crushed when I discovered a pile of supplies stacked on a shiny new baking pan behind the chuckwagon. A tear welled in my eye at their unexpected kindness. Now, it seems I'll be whipping up another batch of those Delights real soon. Good luck with your own bandits, and may they be as considerate as mine.

Chrissy Hartmann

8.2 Colorado Berry Crumble

Serving Size: 3/4 cup
Servings: 6
Approximate Calories: 133

Ingredients:
- 3 cups mixed berries (cranberries, strawberries, blueberries, raspberries)
- 1/4 cup granulated sugar
- 2 tablespoons grapeseed oil
- 1 cup rolled oats
- 1/4 cup all-purpose flour
- 1/4 cup brown sugar
- 1/4 teaspoon salt
- 1/2 teaspoon cinnamon

Instructions:
1. Preheat oven to 350°F.
2. In mixing bowl, combine mixed berries, granulated sugar, and 1 tablespoon of grapeseed oil. Transfer to a baking dish.
3. In another bowl, mix rolled oats, all-purpose flour, brown sugar, salt, cinnamon, and second tablespoon of grapeseed oil.
4. Sprinkle the oat mixture evenly over the berries.
5. Bake for 30-35 minutes or until the crumble is golden and berries are bubbling.
6. Serve warm with vanilla ice cream.

Nutritional Value:
% Daily Value based on a 2000 calorie diet

Total Fat 4.1 g	5%
Saturated Fat 0.5 g	2%
Cholesterol 0 mg	0%
Sodium 2 mg	0%
Carbohydrates 22.7 g	8%
Dietary Fiber 1.7 g	6%
Total Sugars 11.9 g	
Protein 1.8 g	

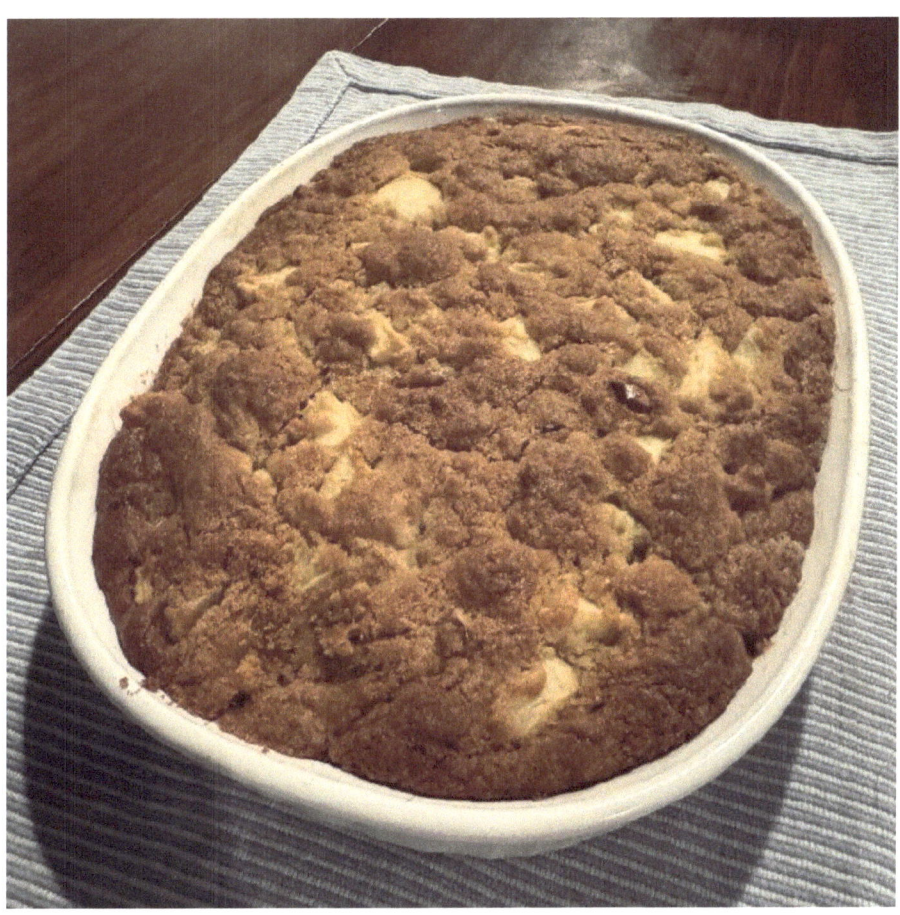

Grumbles from the Chuckwagon:
Big -big thanks from our cowboy family in Colorado. Just wanted to share their recipe, but it comes with a warning. it's a bit of a wilderness wonder — bears seem to have a sweet tooth for it! Last time when we whipped up a batch, left it to cool on the back of the chuckwagon, only to find a bear helping himself to the dish. Apparently, they appreciated the berry crumble as much as we do! So, when baking, keep your eyes peeled for unexpected guests. Enjoy the crumble, just maybe invest in a bear bell for dessert security!
Happy baking,
— Francis Montgomery, Colorado's Finest Chuckwagon Cook

Chrissy Hartmann

8.3 Trails End Banana Bread

Serving Size: 1 slice
Servings: 12
Approximate Calories: 155

Ingredients:
- 3 ripe bananas, mashed
- 1/3 cup grapeseed oil
- 1/2 cup brown sugar
- 1 large egg
- 1 teaspoon pure vanilla extract
- 1 1/2 cups all-purpose flour
- 1/2 teaspoon baking soda
- Optional: 1/2 cup chopped nuts

Instructions:
1. Preheat oven to 350°F. Using a paper towel with a dab of grapeseed oil, Grease the loaf pan.
2. In medium bowl, mix bananas, grapeseed oil, brown sugar, egg, and vanilla extract.
3. In another bowl, sift together to resemble desert sand flour and baking soda.
4. Gradually add dry ingredients to banana mixture and stir until just combined.
5. Fold in chopped nuts if desired.
6. Pour batter into loaf pan and bake for 50-60 minutes or until toothpick comes out clean.
7. Cool in pan, then remove and slice.

Nutritional Value:
% Daily Value based on a 2000 calorie diet
Total Fat 6.7 g   9%
Saturated Fat 0.8 g   4%
Cholesterol 16 mg   5%
Sodium 60 mg   3%
Carbohydrates 22.4 g   8%
Dietary Fiber 0.9 g   3%
Total Sugars 8.4 g
Protein 2.4 g

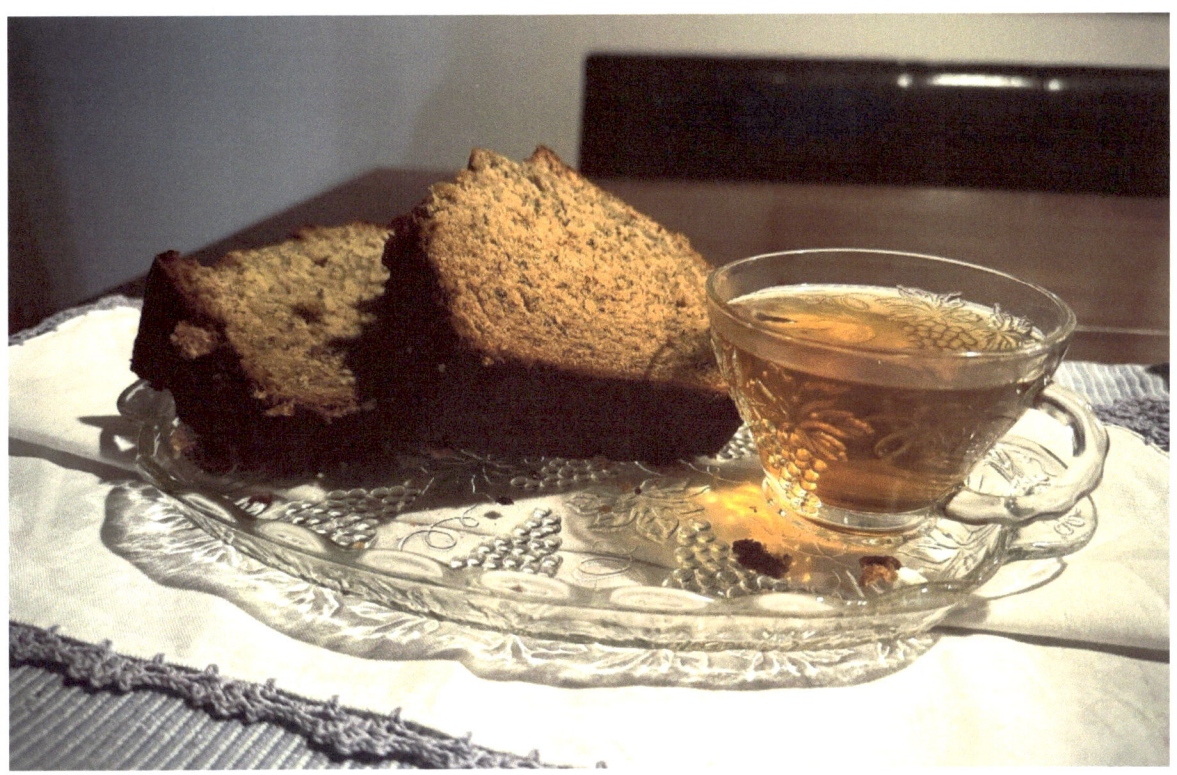

Grumbles from the Chuckwagon:
At trails end, this here bread disappears quick like water sucked up by them desert cacti. So, make two and hide one away. Sometimes I add an extra banana for more flavor if the first three are small. Make sure they are overly ripe. Remember, cowboys aren't afraid to let you know you messed up... at least mine aren't. But if you want to swat that scowl off their face, add some berries for a garnish. It's a sure way to add a little kick to their step.

Chrissy Hartmann

8.4 Apple Cinnamon Cake

Serving Size: 1 slice
Servings: 12
Approximate Calories: 253

Ingredients:
- 2 cups all-purpose flour
- 1 1/2 teaspoons baking powder
- 1/2 teaspoon baking soda
- 1 teaspoon cinnamon
- 1/4 teaspoon salt
- 1/2 cup grapeseed oil
- 1 cup granulated sugar
- 2 large eggs
- 2 teaspoons pure vanilla extract
- 2 cups apples, peeled and diced
- Powdered sugar for dusting

Instructions:
1. Preheat oven to 350°F. Grease and flour baking pan.
2. In bowl, whisk together like a desert sandstorm flour, baking powder, baking soda, cinnamon, and salt.
3. In another bowl, beat grapeseed oil and sugar until well combined.
4. Add eggs and vanilla extract and mix until smooth.
5. Gradually add dry ingredients and fold in the diced apples like a graceful dance partner.
6. Pour batter into prepared pan and bake for 40-45 minutes or until a toothpick comes out clean.
7. Let cake cool, then dust with powdered sugar.
8. Serve warm with ice cream.

Nutritional Value:
% Daily Value based on a 2000 calorie diet

Total Fat 10.2 g	13%
Saturated Fat 1.2 g	6%
Cholesterol 31 mg	10%
Sodium 115 mg	5%
Carbohydrates 38.3 g	14%
Dietary Fiber 1.6 g	6%
Total Sugars 20.8 g	
Protein 3.3 g	

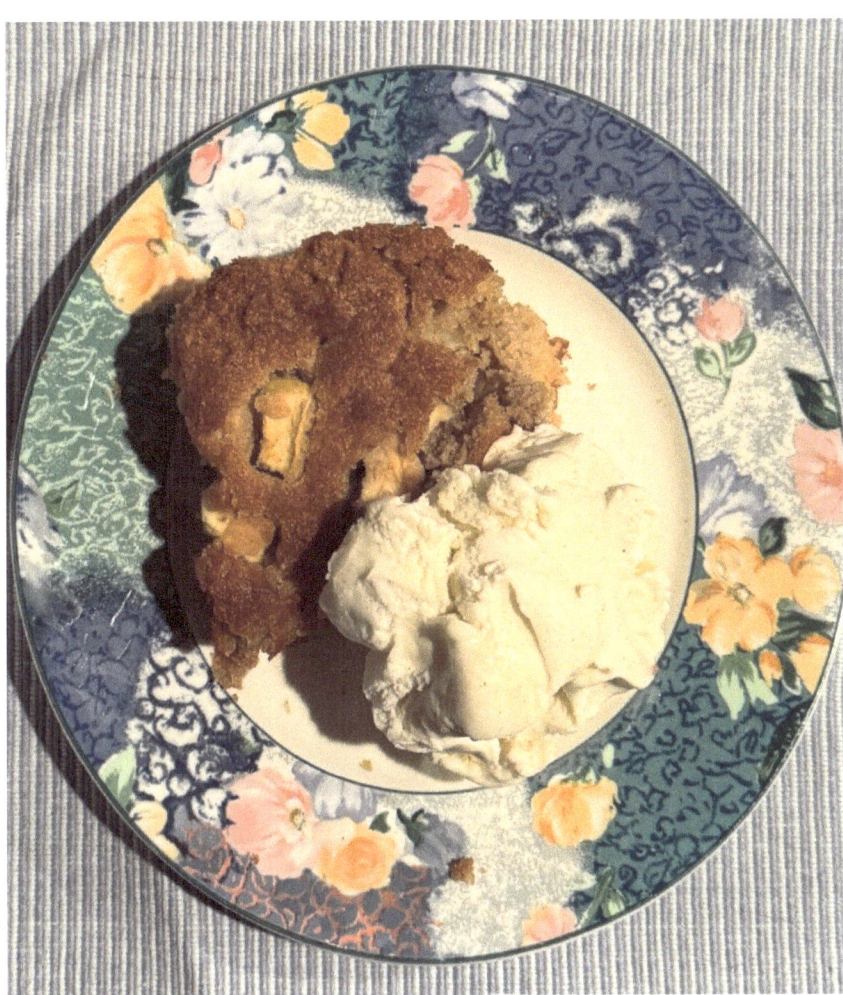

Grumbles from the Chuckwagon:
Now some might think I get advice from a snake oil salesman when it comes to health. but not true. In fact, Old Doc Judd, is the one that told me to eat an apple a day to stay healthy. Don't reckon he meant this way though. But hey, what's a chuckwagon cook supposed to do to get the cowboys to follow Doc's advice? Well, let me tell you, it worked. Hmm? Maybe too well. The fixings seem to show up at the back of the chuckwagon every few days. And by the way, them there golden delicious apples work the best!

Chrissy Hartmann

8.5 Cowboy Cow Chips

Serving Size: 1 cookie
Servings: 24
Approximate Calories: 151

Ingredients:
- 1 cup all-purpose flour
- 1 cup dry oats
- 1/2 cup pumpkin
- 1/2 cup grapeseed oil
- 1/4 teaspoon salt
- 1 teaspoon baking soda
- 3/4 cup granulated sugar
- 3/4 cup brown sugar
- 2 large eggs
- 1 teaspoon pure vanilla extract
- 1 package dark chocolate chips
- 1 package butterscotch chips
- Optional: 1 cup pecan pieces

Instructions:
1. Preheat oven to 350°F. Line baking sheet with parchment paper.
2. In large bowl, whisk together flour, dry oats, baking soda, and salt.
3. In another bowl, mix grapeseed oil, pumpkin, granulated sugar, and brown sugar until smooth.
4. Beat in the eggs and vanilla extract.
5. Gradually add dry ingredients and fold in pecans, dark chocolate and butterscotch chips like a graceful dance partner.
6. Drop spoonfuls of dough onto prepared baking sheet.
7. Bake for 10-12 minutes or until edges are golden.
8. Cool on a wire rack, then serve with milk.

Nutritional Value:
% Daily Value based on a 2000 calorie diet

Total Fat 6.4 g	8%
Saturated Fat 1.4 g	7%
Cholesterol 16 mg	5%
Sodium 82 mg	4%
Carbohydrates 22.6 g	8%
Dietary Fiber 0. 3g	1%

Total Sugars 1 4g
Protein 1.9 g

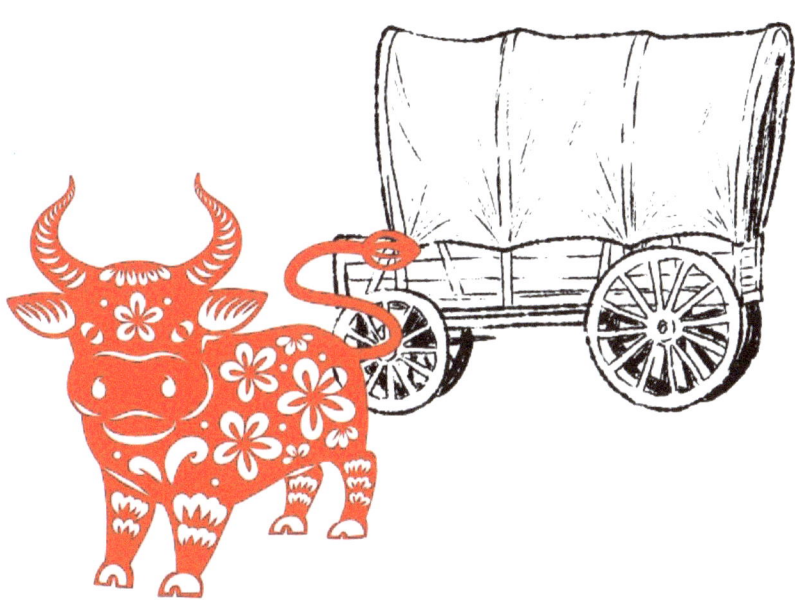

Grumbles from the Chuckwagon:
Oh, sure, just what I need – a grand return to the dusty trail with its enchanting serenade of cattle calls and the sweet melody of spurs. Who wouldn't trade the comfort of this chuckwagon stocked with these here Cowboy Cow Chips and hot brew for the thrill of wrangling, the soothing chorus of hooves, and the enchanting aroma of manure? And don't even get me started on the joy of saddle sores and the gourmet delights of trail dust. Oh, what a paradise it would be to exchange my cozy apron for the lullabies of coyotes and the gentle hum of mosquitoes. As I munch on these cookies, I can practically taste the excitement of herding cattle again in every crumb. Ha! But fear not, for I won't abandon this culinary haven. The chuckwagon is my kingdom, and these Cowboy Cow Chips are my crown jewels. No dusty trail can lure me away from them – not in a million years.

Chrissy Hartmann

8.6 Heavenly Berry Parfait

Servings Size: 1 cup
Servings: 8
Approximate Calories: 214

Ingredients:
- 4 cups mixed berries (strawberries, blueberries, raspberries, cranberries)
- 1/2 cup granola (See chapter 4 for recipe)
- 4 tablespoons honey
- 4 tablespoons grapeseed oil
- 24 ounces Greek yogurt

Instructions:
1. In bowl, combine mixed berries with honey and grapeseed oil.
2. In serving glasses or bowls, layer berry mixture, yogurt, and granola.
3. Repeat layers until glass is filled.
4. Top with a drizzle of honey and a few fresh berries.

Nutritional Value:
% Daily Value based on a 2000 calorie diet

Total Fat 12.4 g	16%
Saturated Fat 2.6 g	13%
Cholesterol 4 mg	1%
Sodium 32 mg	1%
Carbohydrates 28.7 g	10%
Dietary Fiber 3.9 g	14%
Total Sugars 20.1 g	
Protein 11.4 g	

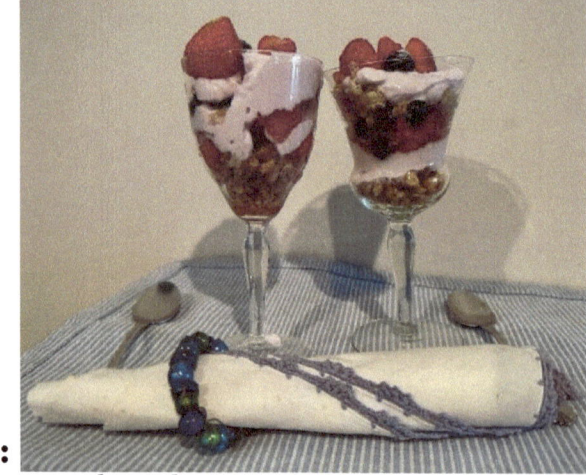

Grumbles from the Chuckwagon:
Okay partner, this is one fancy dessert. Get out your best glassware for this one. It's as pretty as the sunset. I get lots of praise from the cowboys around here for this belly loving dessert. And to let you in on a secret, if the cowboys on your ranch don't like Greek yogurt switch it out for some vanilla pudding. Delicious!

8.7 Toasted Pecan Clusters

Serving Size 1 cluster
Servings: 24
Approximate Calories: 154

Ingredients:
- 3 cups pecans, chopped
- 3/4 cup grapeseed oil
- 1/4 cups brown sugar, packed
- 1/4 cup sugar
- 1 tablespoon ground cinnamon
- 12 ounces dark chocolate, melted

Instructions:
1. Preheat oven to 250°F.
2. In medium mixing bowl combine pecan halves, brown sugar, white sugar, cinnamon, and grapeseed oil, mix well to evenly coat pecan halves.
3. Drop by tablespoon into baking pan.
4. Bake for 20 to 30 minutes, rotate pan halfway through.
5. Remove from pan and place on wax paper, drizzle melted dark chocolate over each cluster.
6. Allow to cool, place in air-tight container to distribute or store.

Nutritional Value:
% daily value based on a 2000 calorie diet

Total Fat 12.3 g	16%
Saturated Fat 2 g	10%
Cholesterol 1 mg	0%
Sodium 4 mg	0%
Carbohydrates 11.8 g	4%
Dietary Fiber 3.7 g	13%
Total Sugars 6.8 g	
Protein 1.8 g	

Grumbles from the Chuckwagon:
From behind the stone countertop, I drizzled dark chocolate over toasted pecans, filling the kitchen with the scent of sweet temptation. The old timers, with faces etched by years on the range, beat the younger cowboys to the clusters, their boots thundering on the floorboards as they raced forward. As the dust settled, victorious whoops filled the air, signaling the timeless triumph of experience over youth. And in that moment, amidst the swirling aroma and the flurry of movement, I knew that some things never change on the cowboy trail.

Chrissy Hartmann

8.8 Lemon Herding Cakes

Serving Size: 1 slice
Servings: 12
Approximate Calories: 127

Ingredients:
- 1 cup all-purpose flour
- 1/2 cup granulated sugar
- 1 teaspoon baking powder
- 1/4 teaspoon salt
- 1/2 cup grapeseed oil
- 2 large eggs
- 1/4 cup fresh lemon juice
- Zest of 1 lemon
- 1/2 teaspoon vanilla extract
- Optional: Powdered sugar, for dusting
- Optional: Fresh berries, for garnish

Instructions:
1. Preheat oven to 350°F. Grease cake pan.
2. In mixing bowl, combine flour, sugar, baking powder, and salt. Mix well.
3. In another bowl, whisk together grapeseed oil, eggs, lemon juice, lemon zest, and vanilla extract until well combined.
4. Gradually add wet ingredients to dry ingredients, stirring until just combined.
5. Pour batter into prepared cake pan, filling about 2/3 full.
6. Bake in preheated oven for 15-17 minutes, or until a toothpick inserted into the center of cake comes out clean.
7. Remove cake from oven and let cool in the pan for 5 minutes before transferring to a wire rack to cool completely.
8. Dust with powdered sugar and serve with fresh berries.

Nutritional Value:
% daily value based on a 2000 calorie diet

Total Fat 6 g	8%
Saturated Fat 1 g	5%
Cholesterol 62 mg	21%
Sodium 838 mg	36%
Carbohydrates 15.1 g	6%
Dietary Fiber 0.4 g	1%
Total Sugars 4.9 g	
Protein 3 g	

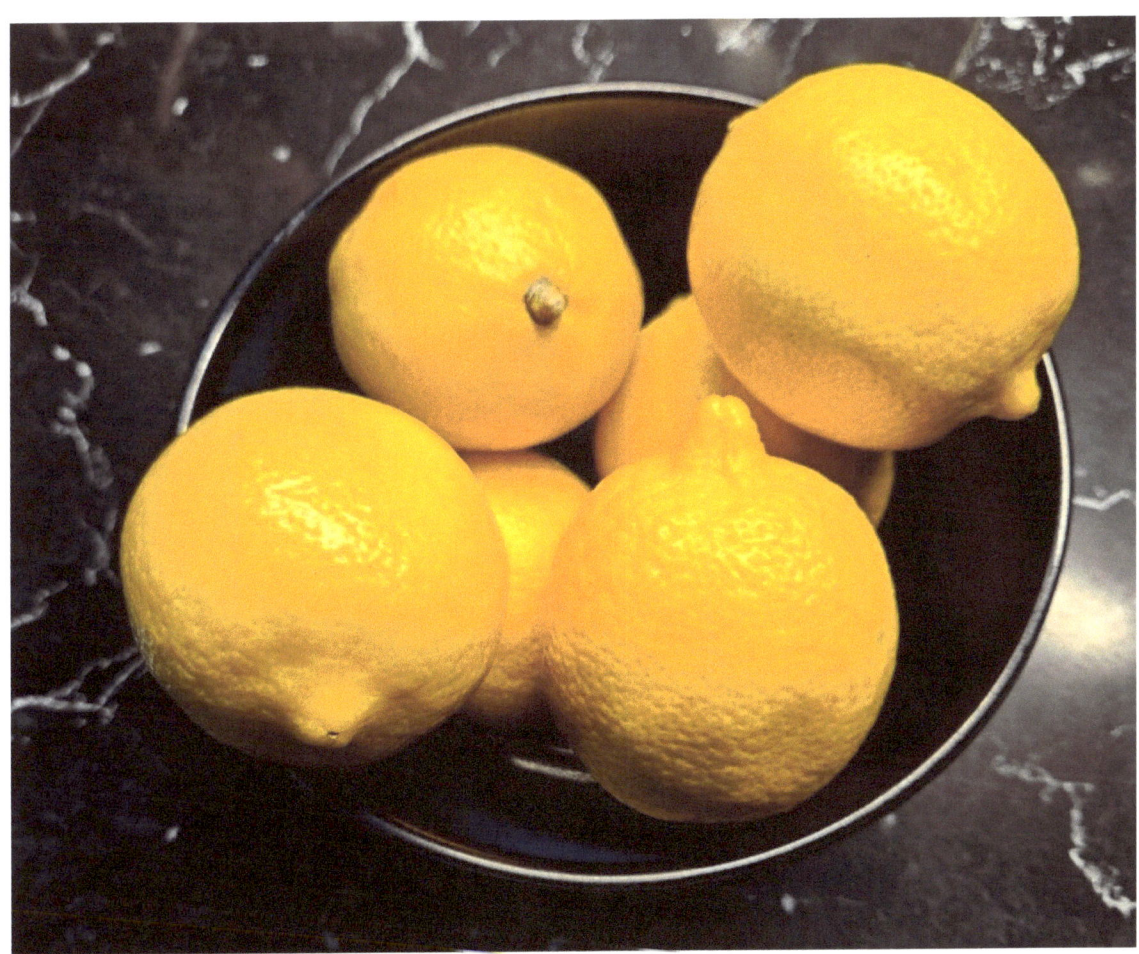

Grumbles from the Chuckwagon:
In the rugged life of managing this chuckwagon, I'm not exactly keen on wrangling fresh lemons. Come dusk, I let slip how the deer were feasting on our lemon trees. Got no rise out of the cowboys, until I hinted we might be at the end of our trail for lemon cakes. Quicker than a twister hits the plains, I'm in the kitchen, potted lemon trees by my side, full basket in hand. Just proves, this seasoned cook knows how to herd the cowboys.

Chrissy Hartmann

8.9 Homestead Pumpkin Funnel Cakes

Serving Size: 1 cake
Servings: 4
Approximate Calories: 650

Ingredients:
- 1/4 cup milk
- 1 egg
- 1 tablespoon water
- 1/2 teaspoon vanilla extract
- 1 tablespoon granulated sugar
- 3/4 teaspoon baking powder
- 1 pinch salt
- 1/2 cup all-purpose flour
- 1/2 cup canned pumpkin
- 4 tablespoons powdered sugar
- Grapeseed oil

Instructions:
1. In a large, spouted bowl, whisk together milk, egg, pumpkin, water, and vanilla.
2. Add sugar, baking powder and salt and whisk until combined.
3. Add the flour and stir until smooth. Set aside.
4. In medium, deep-sided cast iron skillet, heat 1 inch of oil to 375°F over medium-high heat.
5. Reduce heat to medium. Drizzle batter in a thin line, swirling around the pan. Cook for 2 minutes or until light golden brown, then flip and cook another 2 minutes or until golden brown.
6. Remove with tongs and dust with 2 tablespoons powdered sugar and serve.
7. Repeat steps 1-6 with the remaining batter.

Nutritional Value:
% Daily Value based on a 2000 calorie diet

Total Fat 11.3 g	14%
Saturated Fat 1.7 g	9%
Cholesterol 94 mg	31%
Sodium 9747 mg	424%
Carbohydrates 146 g	53%
Dietary Fiber 1.1 g	4%
Total Sugars 125.4 g	
Protein 48 g	

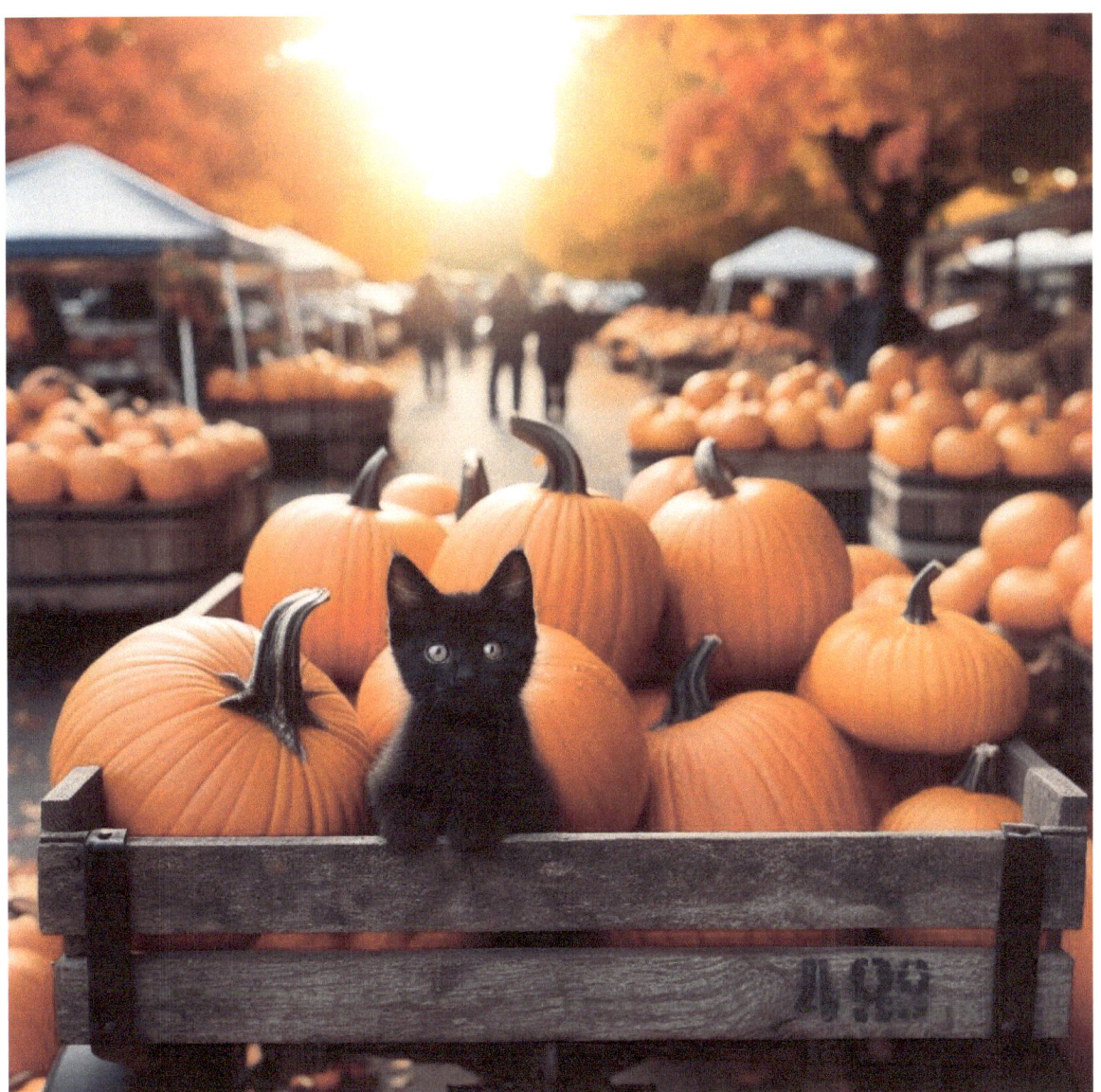

Grumbles from the Chuckwagon:
Want to make a cowboy smile? Whether it be from the kitchen or chuckwagon, just serve them up one of these here pumpkin funnel cakes. It will remind them of those carefree days at the county fair when their teeth sink into the crisp dough, and they taste the sweet pumpkin . Their eyes will sparkle with delight, and you may even garner a kiss of thanks or two... for the memories... not that any cowboy kissed me. But, my cowgirl? That's a different tale.

Chrissy Hartmann

8.10 Peanut Brittle

Serving Size: 1
Servings: 20+
Approximate Calories: 131

Ingredients:
- 1 cup granulated sugar
- 1/2 cup light corn syrup
- 1/4 cup water
- 1 cup raw peanuts (unsalted)
- 2 tablespoons grapeseed oil
- 1 teaspoon vanilla extract
- 1 teaspoon baking soda
- A pinch of salt

Instructions:
1. Line baking sheet with parchment paper. Set aside.
2. In heavy-bottomed saucepan, combine granulated sugar, corn syrup, and water. Cook over medium heat, stirring constantly, until the sugar has dissolved.
3. Once sugar has dissolved, add the raw peanuts to the saucepan. Continue cooking, stirring frequently, until mixture reaches temperature of 300°F on candy thermometer. This is the hard crack stage.
4. Remove saucepan from heat. Quickly stir in grapeseed oil and vanilla extract until well incorporated into the mixture.
5. Sprinkle baking soda and a pinch of salt over mixture, then quickly stir to combine. Be careful, as mixture will bubble up when you add baking soda.
6. Immediately pour hot peanut brittle mixture onto lined baking sheet. Use spatula to spread out into an even layer, about 1/4 inch thick.
7. Allow peanut brittle to cool completely at room temperature, about 1 hour. Once cooled, break into pieces using knife.
8. Store peanut brittle in an airtight container at room temperature for up to 2 weeks. Enjoy!

Nutritional Value:
% Daily Value based on a 2000 calorie diet

Total Fat 10.4 g	13%
Saturated Fat 1.1 g	5%
Cholesterol 0 mg	0%
Sodium 1142 mg	50%
Carbohydrates 7 g	3%
Dietary Fiber 0.4 g	1%
Total Sugars 5.4 g	
Protein 1.1 g	

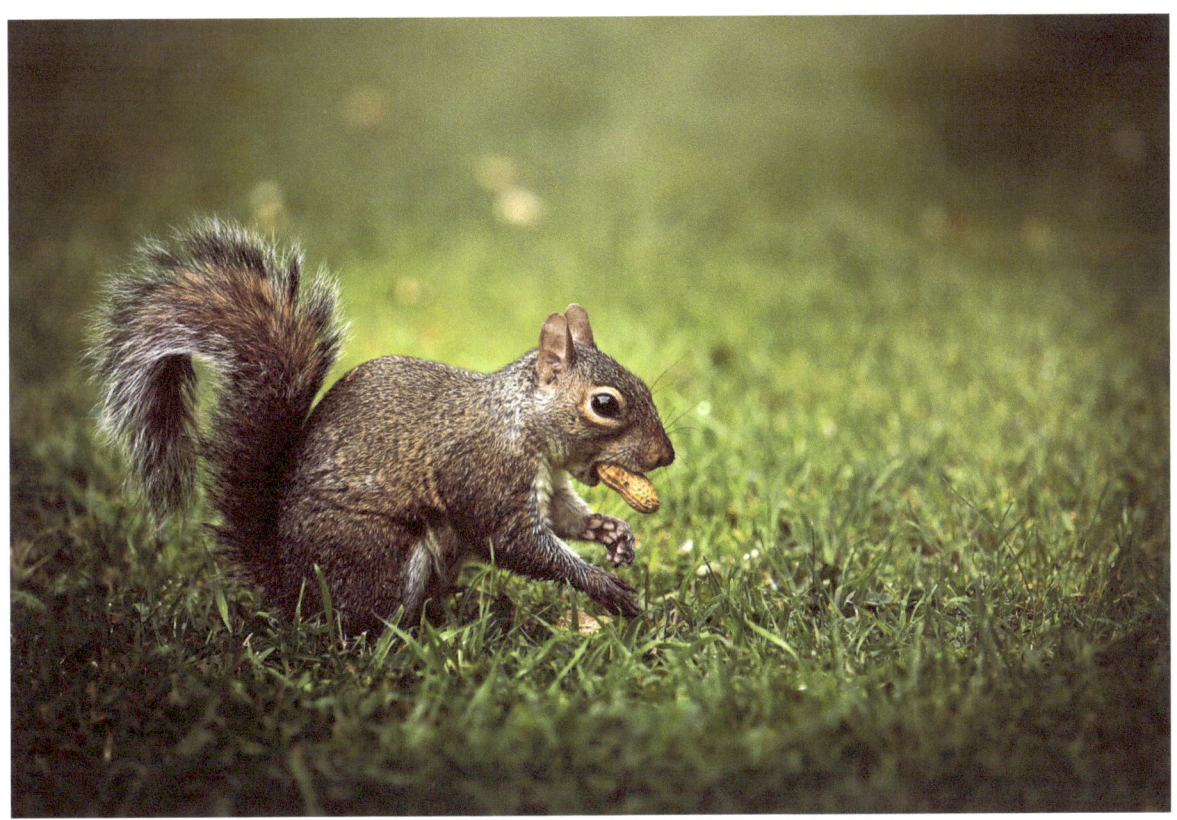

Grumbles from the Chuckwagon :
Not your typical dessert, but when the cowboys want a little something sweet to crunch on, they don't squirrel around. They'll lasso the chance for some of this here peanut brittle. It provides a quick energy-boost during long days on the trail or at the rodeo.

Chrissy Hartmann

8.11 Texas Carrot Cake

Serving Size: 1
Servings: 16
Approximate Calories: 552

Ingredients:
- 1-1/4 cups grapeseed oil
- 2 cups granulated sugar
- 3 eggs room temperature
- 2 cups all-purpose flour
- 1 teaspoon baking soda
- 1-1/2 teaspoon baking powder
- 1/2 teaspoon salt
- 1 teaspoon cinnamon
- 2 cups grated carrots
- 1 cup chopped pecans
- 1 teaspoon vanilla

Ingredients Cream Cheese Frosting:
- 4 cups powdered sugar
- 8 ounces cream cheese, softened
- 1 teaspoon vanilla

Instructions:
1. Preheat oven to 350°F. Lightly grease and flour 9×13 pan.
2. Combine grapeseed oil, vanilla, sugar, and eggs in large bowl. Then Add flour, baking soda, baking powder, salt, and cinnamon. Stir well. Then fold in carrots and pecans.
3. Pour into pan, bake 35-40 minutes.
4. While cake bakes, mix in small bowl cream cheese frosting ingredients.
5. Let cake cool 10 minutes then frost and top with toasted pecans.

Nutritional Value:
% Daily Value based on a 2000 calorie diet

Total Fat 30.3 g	39%
Saturated Fat 12.7 g	63%
Cholesterol 125 mg	42%
Sodium 314 mg	135%
Carbohydrates 60.1 g	22%
Dietary Fiber 4.8 g	17%
Total Sugars 39.8 g	
Protein 8.5 g	

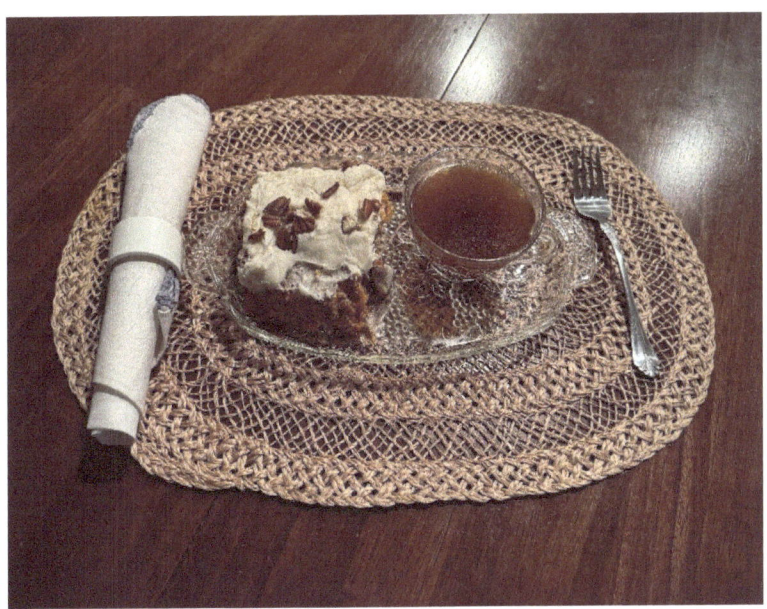

Grumbles from the Chuckwagon:
Now here's a Texas carrot cake that's downright delicious, but let me warn ya, it's rich in calories. Perfect for celebrating something special, but watch your meal planning for the day., I've used grapeseed oil, so it leans toward the heart-healthy side. Just remember, a little slice goes a long way - enjoy in moderation. And hey, maybe take an extra lap or two around the pasture today... without your horse!

Chrissy Hartmann

8.12 Cowboy Cookies

Serving Size: 1 cookie
Servings: 24
Calories: 91

Ingredients:
- 1-1/2 cups all-purpose flour
- 1/2 tablespoon baking powder
- 1/2 tablespoon baking soda
- Optional: 1/2 tablespoon cinnamon
- 1/2 teaspoon salt
- 1 cup grapeseed oil
- 3/4 cups sugar
- 3/4 2 cups brown sugar packed
- 2 eggs
- 1/2 tablespoon pure vanilla extract
- 1-1/2 cups dark chocolate morsels
- Optional: 1-1/2 cups butterscotch morsels
- 1-1/2 cups old- fashioned rolled oats
- 1 cup sweet coconut flakes
- 1 cups chopped pecan halves

Instructions:
1. Preheat oven to 350°F.
2. Sift to resemble desert sand in a large bowl flour, baking powder, baking soda, salt, and cinnamon.
3. mix grapeseed oil, vanilla extract, and sugars until smooth.
4. Add eggs, one at a time.
5. Stir in flour mixture, after thoroughly mixed, blend in oats, chocolate chips, pecans, and coconut.
6. Drop dough onto the ungreased cookie sheet by tablespoon.
7. Bake for 11 – 13 minutes, rotate cookie sheets half-way through. Remove from oven, let cool for a few minutes then place on cooling rack.

Nutritional Value:
% daily value based on a 2000 calorie diet

Total Fat 8.9 g	11%
Saturated Fat 1. 9 g	10%
Cholesterol 23 mg	8%
Sodium 1388 mg	60%
Carbohydrates 22.9 g	8%
Dietary Fiber 2.4 g	9%
Total Sugars 10.1 g	
Protein 3.2 g	

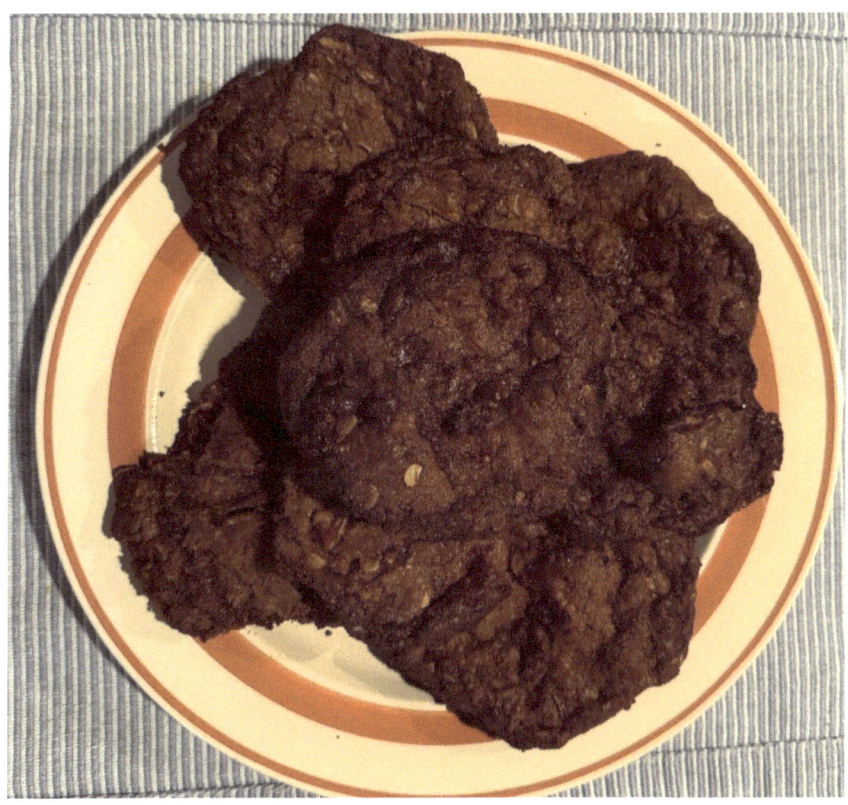

Grumbles from the Chuckwagon:
Now here's the blue-ribbon winner of cookies. Huge as Texas, these here heart healthy cookies are packed with grapeseed oil and oats combined with dark chocolate, sweet coconut, and cinnamon. When the boys don't have time to eat, they grab a few of these here cookies to tide the hunger pains. One is plenty, but two is better. So, cowboy up and lasso yourself a couple. You'll finish them quicker than 8 seconds flat.

Chrissy Hartmann

The Grub Wrangler's Wisdom:

Chapter 9 Dressings, Drizzles, and more

Howdy, culinary cowpokes! Welcome to the roundup of flavors in our chapter of dressings and more. And boy howdy, do we have more!

Now, in the wild west of the kitchen, we've got dressings that'll lasso your salads into submission, drizzles that'll make your taste buds two-step, and sauces that'll have you wishing for more. And remember, each one's a taste adventure, ripe for tweaking to suit your liking.

Now, gather 'round for a tale about how we whipped up the Homemade Mayo. Them chickens, crafty critters, had been rustling their own eggs. Caught them red-handed in the barn, clucking and conspiring. Figured we'd turn the tables – made that mayo so tasty with that liquid gold of grapeseed oil, even the chickens couldn't resist. Moral of the story: even culinary outlaws can turn a coop catastrophe into a kitchen triumph. So, saddle up, flavor seekers, and let's rustle up some culinary

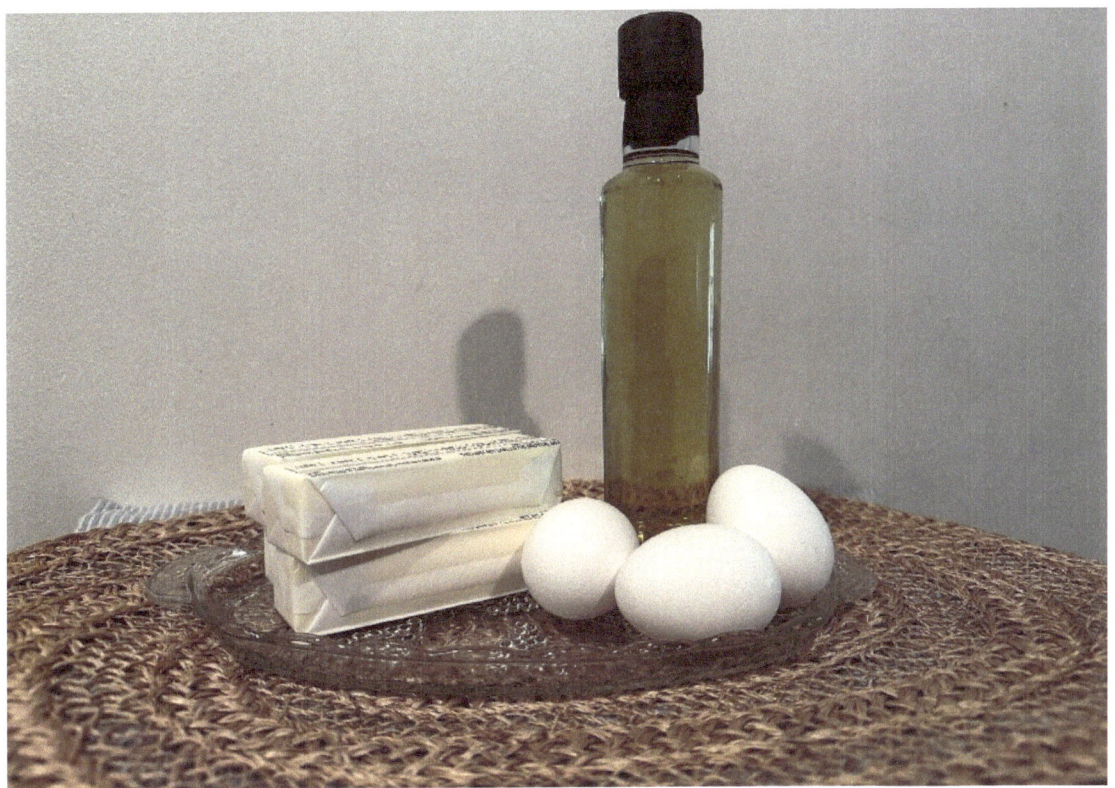

Chrissy Hartmann

9.1 Classic Balsamic Vinaigrette

Serving Size: 1 Tablespoon
Servings: 16
Approximate Calories: 123

Ingredients:
- 1 cup grapeseed oil
- 3/4 cup balsamic vinegar
- 3 teaspoon Dijon mustard
- Salt and pepper to taste

Instructions:
1. Whisk all ingredients together in a bowl until well combined.
2. Drizzle over your favorite salad.
3. Store unused portion in refrigerator.

Nutritional Value:
% Daily Value based on a 2000 calorie diet

Total Fat 13.7 g	18%
Saturated Fat 1.3 g	7%
Cholesterol 0 mg	0%
Sodium 11 mg	0%
Carbohydrates 0.3 g	0%
Dietary Fiber 0 g	0%
Total Sugars 0 g	
Protein 0.1 g	

Grumbles from the Chuckwagon:
Ever have trouble getting your cowboy to eat a salad? Try this one. It's light and lets the flavor of your veggies shine through like sun rays on a field of wildflowers. And it helps keep the body fit inside and out. But if their inner-yellow belly starts to whine about eating salads, then drizzle this over some green beans wrapped in bacon.

9.2 Lemon-Honey Dijon Dressing

Serving Size: 1 Tablespoon
Servings: 16
Approximate Calories: 127

Ingredients:
- 1 cup grapeseed oil
- 1/2 cup fresh lemon juice
- 4 tablespoon honey
- 1 Tablespoon Dijon mustard
- Salt and pepper to taste

Instructions:
1. Whisk the ingredients together until the dressing is smooth.
2. Use it on mixed greens or as a marinade for chicken.
3. Store in refrigerator.

Nutritional Value:
% Daily Value based on a 2000 calorie diet

Total Fat 13.7 g	18%
Saturated Fat 1.4 g	7%
Cholesterol 0 mg	0%
Sodium 13 mg	1%
Carbohydrates 1.3 g	0%
Dietary Fiber 0.1 g	0%
Total Sugars 1.3 g	
Protein 0.1 g	

Grumbles from the Chuckwagon:
This here dressing gets high praise from the cowboys. When the chuckwagon serves up grilled chicken, we have to make a double batch. It's also a blue-ribbon winner for salads. The light tang of the lemon and mustard and sweetness of the honey blend together like a gentle stream with the grapeseed oil. It's mouth-watering delicious!

Chrissy Hartmann

9.3 Sesame Dressing:

Servings Size: 1 Tablespoon
Servings: 16
Approximate Calories: 143

Ingredients:
- 1 cup grapeseed oil
- 4 tablespoons rice vinegar
- 2 tablespoon soy sauce
- 2 tablespoon sesame oil
- 2 teaspoon honey
- 2 clove garlic, minced
- 1 teaspoon grated ginger

Instructions:
1. Whisk all ingredients together until well combined.
2. Drizzle over an Asian-inspired salad or use as a marinade for grilled tofu.
3. Refrigerate when not using.

Nutritional Value:
% Daily Value based on a 2000 calorie diet

Total Fat 15.3 g	20%
Saturated Fat 1.6 g	8%
Cholesterol 0 mg	0%
Sodium 113 mg	5%
Carbohydrates 1.1 g	0%
Dietary Fiber 0 g	0%
Total Sugars 0.8 g	
Protein 0.2 g	

Grumbles from the Chuckwagon:
Unfortunately, this is as far east my cowboys will go. they'll will actually eat a tofu salad with this dressing. Don't even have to get out the rope to hog tie them to the table. Yeehaw!

9.4 Sweet Orange Dressing

Serving Size: 1 Tablespoon
Servings: 16
Approximate Calories: 138

Ingredients:
- 1 cup grapeseed oil
- 1/2 cup orange juice
- 3 tablespoon honey
- Zest of 2 oranges
- Salt to taste

Instructions:
1. Whisk together ingredients in a bowl.
2. Drizzle over spinach and strawberry salad or chicken stir fry.
3. Refrigerate when not in use.

Nutritional Value:
% Daily Value based on a 2000 calorie diet

Total Fat 13. mg	18%
Saturated Fat 1.3 g	7%
Cholesterol 0 mg	0%
Sodium 0 mg	0%
Carbohydrates 4.2 g	2%
Dietary Fiber 0.1 g	0%
Total Sugars 4 g	
Protein 0.2 g	

Grumbles from the Chuckwagon:
This here sweet orange dressing over chicken stir fry sometimes brings on a shootout quicker than the boys from the Okay Corral if we run out. And let's not even discuss what happens when it's served on a grilled chicken salad. I reckon you might double up the batch.

Chrissy Hartmann

9.5 Raspberry-Lime Vinaigrette

Serving Size: 1 Tablespoon
Servings: 16
Approximate Calories: 149

Ingredients:
- 1 cup grapeseed oil
- 1/2 cup fresh lime juice
- 1/2 cup raspberry preserves
- 1-1/2 teaspoon Dijon mustard
- Salt and pepper to taste

Instructions:
1. Mix all ingredients together until smooth.
2. Drizzle over a mixed berry and goat cheese salad or switch out the lime for lemon and brush on salmon.
3. Refrigerate when finished.

Nutritional Value:
% Daily Value based on a 2000 calorie diet

Total Fat 13.7 g	18%
Saturated Fat 1.3 g	7%
Cholesterol 0 mg	0%
Sodium 7 mg	0%
Carbohydrates 6.9 g	3%
Dietary Fiber 0.1 g	0%
Total Sugars 4.9 g	
Protein 0.1 g	

Grumbles from the Chuckwagon:
   For the cowgirl ladies... A definite favorite. Lime and raspberry dressing that dances on your tongue like a real hoedown. You'll be kicking up your heels and swirling your skirt with this one. And let's not forget the cowboys. Mine love it on chicken. Their taste buds will love you for this.

9.6 Maple-Dijon Glaze

Serving Size: 1 Tablespoon
Servings: 16
Calories: 150

Ingredients:
- 1 cup grapeseed oil
- 1/2 cup maple syrup
- 4 tablespoon Dijon mustard
- 2 - 3 clove garlic, minced
- Salt and pepper to taste

Instructions:
1. Whisk all the ingredients until the glaze is well combined.
2. Use it to glaze roasted vegetables or grilled salmon.
3. Store in refrigerator.

Nutritional Value:
% Daily Value based on a 2000 calorie diet

Total Fat 13.8 g	18%
Saturated Fat 1.3 g	7%
Cholesterol 0 mg	0%
Sodium 45 mg	2%
Carbohydrates 7 g	3%
Dietary Fiber 0.1 g	1%
Total Sugars 5.9 g	
Protein 0.2 g	

Grumbles from the Chuckwagon:
A bronco buster for veggies! Woohoo! Big Texas thanks to a very special cowboy who donated this recipe to our cookbook. If you use a lot like we do on our veggies, try using our brown sugar syrup instead, tastes just like maple syrup. You'll never have to rob another bank again to replenish your stock. Did we say, "Woohoo?"

Chrissy Hartmann

9.7 Honey Mustard Glaze

Serving Size: 1 Tablespoon
Servings: 16
Approximate Calories: 153

Ingredients:
- 1 cup grapeseed oil
- 1/2 cup honey
- 1/2 cup whole-grain mustard
- 2 cloves garlic, minced
- Salt and pepper to taste

Instructions:
1. Whisk together ingredients until the glaze is smooth.
2. Brush it over grilled chicken or drizzle on roasted Brussels sprouts.
3. Store in refrigerator when not using.

Nutritional Value:
% Daily Value based on a 2000 calorie diet

Total Fat 13.6 g	17%
Saturated Fat 1.3 g	7%
Cholesterol 0 mg	0%
Sodium 0 mg	0%
Carbohydrates 8.9 g	3%
Dietary Fiber 0 g	0%
Total Sugars 8.7 g	
Protein 0.1 g	

Grumbles from the Chuckwagon:
Zesty yet sweet. The chicken and veggies don't stand a chance with this glaze. Simple and easy to make and that's what my cowboys appreciate. Yes, that means if they can make it anyone can. And if you want it to kick like a wild bronco for chicken, shrimp, salmon, or beef, add chili powder. Yeehaw!

9.8 Sweet-N-Sour Dressing

Serving Size: 1 Tablespoon
Servings: 16
Approximate Calories: 154

Ingredients:
- 1 cup grapeseed oil
- ⅔ cup white sugar
- ⅓ cup distilled white vinegar
- ¼ small onion, finely diced
- 1 teaspoon salt
- ¾ teaspoon dry mustard
- ½ teaspoon celery seed

Instructions:
1. In a bowl combine dry ingredients and mix evenly.
2. Add distilled white vinegar.
3. Mix in grapeseed oil stirring it evenly (If too thick add 1 tsp of water until desired thickness).
4. Drizzle over grilled chicken salad, stir fry, or use in pasta salad.

Nutritional Value:
% Daily Value based on a 2000 calorie diet

Total Fat 13.7 g	18%
Saturated Fat 1.3 g	7%
Cholesterol 0 mg	0%
Sodium 0 mg	0%
Carbohydrates 8.5 g	3%
Dietary Fiber 0 g	0%
Total Sugars 8.4 g	
Protein 0.1 g	

Grumbles from the Chuckwagon:
We here on the ranch love this dressing. In fact we use it not only on salads, but chicken. It's fabulous mixing it with our vinaigrette for pasta salad. Your taste buds will shoot to the stars after tasting this one.

Chrissy Hartmann

9.9 Homemade Mayonnaise

Serving Size: 1 Tablespoon
Servings: 1 cup
Approximate Calories: 129

Ingredients:
- 2 Large eggs, room temperature
- 2 Teaspoons fresh squeezed lemon juice (or vinegar)
- 1 Cup Grapeseed oil
- A pinch of fine grain sea salt

Instructions:
1. Separate egg whites from yolks. Set aside egg whites for another purpose.
2. Pour fresh lemon juice (or vinegar) into bowl with the egg yolks and whisk them well.
3. pour oil into bowl a few drops at a time while whisking constantly. Once mayonnaise has started to thicken, pour oil in a slow and steady stream. If oil starts to build up at all, stop pouring and whisk mayonnaise briskly until oil has incorporated.
4. Season it carefully with fine grain sea salt. Add a small splash of water if you would like a thinner mayonnaise, about 1 teaspoon at a time.

Nutritional Value:
% Daily Value based on a 2000 calorie diet

Total Fat 14.3 g	18%
Saturated Fat 1.5 g	8%
Cholesterol 23 mg	8%
Sodium 9 mg	0%
Carbohydrates 0.1 g	0%
Dietary Fiber 0 g	0%
Total Sugars 0.1 g	
Protein 0.8 g	

Grumbles from the Chuckwagon:
The cowboys around here love the homemade fixings. So why not make a mayo that's good for the heart too? All natural and no preservatives. Light, fresh, and tasty when added to salads or sandwiches.

9.10 Chipotle Drizzle

Serving Size: 1 Tablespoon
Servings: 24
Approximate Calories: 175

Ingredients:
- 1 cup grapeseed oil
- 1/2 cup red wine vinegar
- 1 teaspoon cumin
- 1/2 teaspoon chili powder
- 2 clove garlic minced
- 2 tablespoon honey
- Pinch of salt and pepper

Instructions:
1. In a bowl combine dry ingredients and mix evenly.
2. Add distilled white vinegar and honey.
3. Mix in grapeseed oil stirring it evenly (If too thick add 1 tsp of water until desired thickness).
4. Drizzle or brush over veggies, salads, steak, fish, or chicken.
5. Store in refrigerator when not in use.

Nutritional Value:
% Daily Value based on a 2000 calorie diet
Total Fat 18.2 g	23%
Saturated Fat 1.7 g	9%
Cholesterol 0 mg	0%
Sodium 2 mg	0%
Carbohydrates 3.3 g	1%
Dietary Fiber 0.1 g	0%
Total Sugars 2.9 g	
Protein 0.1 g	

Grumbles from the Chuckwagon:
Who needs to run for the border when we can make our own Mexican cuisine here at the chuckwagon. Fabulous on Chicken fish, or steak!

Chrissy Hartmann

9.11 Honey Barbecue Sauce

Serving Size: 1 Tablespoon
Servings: 32
Approximate Calories: 47

Ingredients:
- 1 cup ketchup
- 1/2 cup grapeseed oil
- 1/4 cup apple cider vinegar
- 1/4 cup honey
- 2 tablespoons Worcestershire sauce
- 1 tablespoon Dijon mustard
- 1 teaspoon smoked paprika
- 1 teaspoon garlic powder
- Salt and pepper to taste
- Optional: Liquid smoke to taste

Instructions:
1. Combine in a medium sized bowl.
2. Stir briskly until well blended. If sauce is too thick, add 1 tablespoon of water for desired thickness.
3. Coat desired meat on grill making sure to turn occasionally after reapplying.
4. Store in refrigerator when not in use.

Nutritional Value:
% daily value based on a 2000 calorie diet

Total Fat 2.1 g	3%
Saturated Fat 0.2 g	1%
Cholesterol 0 mg	0%
Sodium 141 mg	6%
Carbohydrates 6.9 g	3%
Dietary Fiber 1.6 g	6%
Total Sugars 3.7 g	
Protein 1.2 g	

Grumbles from the Chuckwagon:
Perfect for grilling. Zesty, sweet taste that your cowboy will come back for more. And if you got any of them there little cowpokes running around, they'll love dipping their chicken nuggets in it too. Can't keep it in stock. My Cowboys love it!

9.12 Spicy Vidalia Sauce

Serving Size: 1 tablespoon
Servings: 16
Approximate Calories: 139

Ingredients:
- 1 medium-or 1/2 large size Vidalia Onion, finely chopped
- 1 cup ketchup
- 2 tablespoons firmly packed brown sugar
- 2 tablespoons fresh lemon juice
- 2 tablespoons apple cider vinegar
- 2 tablespoons Worcestershire sauce
- 1 tablespoon grapeseed oil
- 1 garlic clove, minced
- 1/2 teaspoon salt
- 1/2 teaspoon Pepper

Instructions:
1. Combine all ingredients into a large saucepan.
2. Add 1 cup of water.
3. Bring to a boil over medium heat.
4. Reduce heat to low, and simmer for 20 minutes, stirring occasionally.
5. When cool, use as desired. Refrigerate when not in use.

Nutritional Value:
% daily value based on a 2000 calorie diet

Total Fat 6.5 g	8%
Saturated Fat 0.7 g	4%
Cholesterol 0 mg	0%
Sodium 1360 mg	59%
Carbohydrates 19.5 g	7%
Dietary Fiber 1.1 g	4%
Total Sugars 15.2 g	
Protein 0.9 g	

Grumbles from the Chuckwagon:
Want to add that extra sweet kick to your dish? This here is the sauce to do it. Great twist to stuffed mushrooms or that burger with bacon. It's a sauce that will liven up any ghost town of a dish. Yeehaw!

Chrissy Hartmann

9.13 Lemon Cream Sauce

Serving Size: 1 tablespoon
Servings: 6
Approximate Calories: 190

Ingredients:
    1 cup dry vermouth
- 1 cup heavy whipping cream
- 4 tablespoons grapeseed oil
- 2 tablespoons lemon juice
- 1 tablespoon fresh lemon zest
- salt and pepper to taste

Instructions:
1. Reduce dry vermouth in a small saucepan, set over medium heat.
2. Once reduced, add cream and cook until slightly thickened.
3. Then stir in the lemon juice.
4. Simmer until the sauce has thickened slightly then remove from the heat.
5. Whisk in the grapeseed oil , adding one tablespoon at a time, until thickened and smooth.
6. Season to taste with salt and pepper and serve.

Nutritional Value:
% Daily value based on a 2000 calorie diet

Total Fat 73.1 g	94%
Saturated Fat 10.5 g	53%
Cholesterol 23 mg	8%
Sodium 13 mg	1%
Carbohydrates 1.7 g	1%
Dietary Fiber 0.1 g	0%
Total Sugars 0.7 g	

Grumbles from the Chuckwagon:
I slathered the creamy lemon sauce onto the blackened catfish, feeling a bit proud watching that rich layer set against the char. As the cowboys dug in, their jaws slowed, savoring that first bite. One of 'em looked up, smacking his lips. "Gus, what'd you put in this?"
"Little lemon, little cream," I shrugged. "Keeps things interesting."
The cowboy wiped his mouth, a sly grin spreading. "You keep making that sauce, we'll catch as many catfish as you need."

9.14 Plum Delicious Ginger Dipping Sauce

Serving Size: 1 tablespoon
Servings : 6
Approximate Calories: 190

Ingredients:
- 1 teaspoon grapeseed oil
- 3 plums, firm.
- 2 teaspoon fresh ginger, peeled and minced
- 2 cloves garlic, minced
- 1 cup low-sodium chicken broth
- 1 tablespoon honey

Instructions:
1. Over medium heat, cook the pitted and diced plums with the grapeseed oil and ginger. Stir occasionally for 3 minutes.
2. Add the garlic and cook, stir often for 2 minutes.
3. Add broth.
4. Cover saucepan, cook for 4 minutes.
5. Remove lid and continue cooking until sauce reduces and plums soften, about 5 to 10 minutes.
6. Stir in honey and simmer another 1-2 minutes.
7. Chill before dipping, enjoy!
8. Store unused portion in refrigerator.

Nutritional Value:
% daily value based on a 2000 calorie diet

Total Fat 28.4 g	36%
Saturated Fat 3.4 g	17%
Cholesterol 0 mg	0%
Sodium 33 mg	1%
Carbohydrates 78.6 g	29%
Dietary Fiber 8 g	29%
Total Sugars 28 g	
Protein 8.4 g	

Grumbles from the Chuckwagon:
Now this here chuckwagon don't get plums that often. When we do, those critters are made up into this plum sauce. That's right, they don't last long when word gets out. So that everyone gets a taste, we stoke up the campfire and cook up a batch of sauce. Best thing I've ever done to get these here cowboys eating healthy. Heck, we now have to double up on our order of vegetables when the plums are in season. It's just plum delicious!

Chrissy Hartmann

The Grub Wrangler's Wisdom:

Chapter 10 Cooking and Baking Tips

Well, Partner, reckon you made it to chapter 10 and these here recipes are setting your taste buds on a two-step hoedown, right? So, before you mosey on, , though don't forget to tip your hat to these here cooking and baking nuggets about using grapeseed oil. They are the secret ingredients to wrangling up flavors that will leave you wanting more.

Remember even though, grapeseed oil has many advantages, it's still important to consider the specific requirements and characteristics of your recipes to achieve the best results. Additionally, be aware of any potential allergens if you or your guests have allergies to grape products.

So don't ride off into the sunset yet, Let's rustle up some culinary magic with these here tricks.

Happy cooking and may your kitchen be as lively as a country fair hoedown .

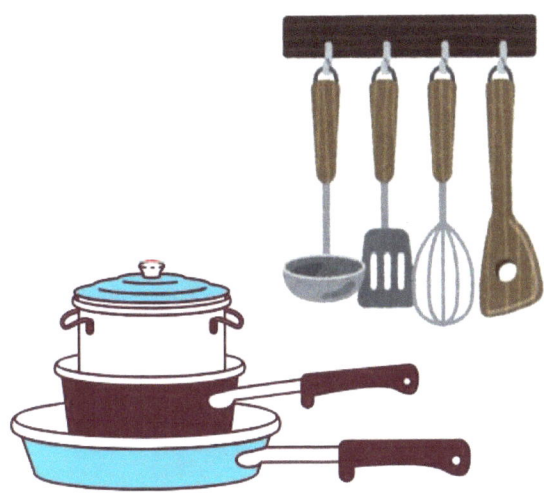

Chrissy Hartmann

10.1 Cooking Tips

1. High Smoke Point: Grapeseed oil has a high smoke point, making it suitable for high-heat cooking methods like grilling, frying, sautéing, and stir-frying. It won't break down or produce harmful compounds at high temperatures.

2. Neutral Flavor: Grapeseed oil has a mild, neutral flavor that won't overpower the taste of your dishes. It's an excellent choice when you want the natural flavors of your ingredients to shine.

3. Light Texture: This oil has a light and clean texture, making it ideal for salad dressings, marinades, and as a finishing oil.

4. Heart-Healthy: Grapeseed oil is rich in unsaturated fats, particularly monounsaturated fats and polyunsaturated fats, which can be beneficial for heart health.

5. Use for Roasting: Its high smoke point makes it perfect for roasting vegetables, ensuring they maintain a crisp texture and natural flavors.

6. Replacing Butter: When sautéing or roasting, consider using grapeseed oil as a healthier alternative to butter. It reduces saturated fat intake.

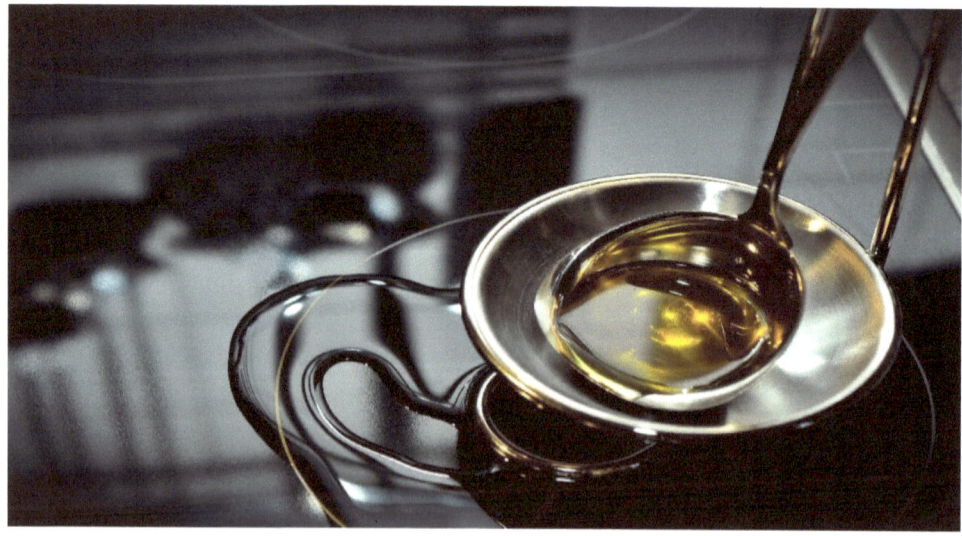

10.2 Baking Tips

1. Substitute for Butter: You can often substitute grapeseed oil for butter in baking recipes. Use a 1:1 ratio but remember that the texture and flavor of your baked goods may differ slightly.

2. Muffin and Quick Bread Moisture: Grapeseed oil adds moisture to muffins and quick bread, resulting in a softer crumb. Use it as a healthier option.

3. Cakes: When using grapeseed oil in cakes, whisk it with the sugar to incorporate air, ensuring a light and fluffy texture.

4. Milder Flavor: Grapeseed oil's neutral taste makes it suitable for cakes and cookies when you want a milder oil flavor.

5. Nutrient Retention: Grapeseed oil's high smoke point helps preserve the nutritional content of baked goods.

6. Uniform Mixing: When using grapeseed oil in your baking, mix it thoroughly with other wet ingredients to ensure an even distribution of fats throughout the batter.

7. Monitor Temperature: If a recipe calls for a specific fat to be melted, like butter, you may need to slightly adjust the baking temperature when using grapeseed oil to avoid over-browning.

8. Be Mindful of Texture: Keep in mind that grapeseed oil can make baked goods slightly denser than butter, so it may not be the best choice for every recipe.

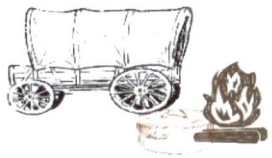

Chrissy Hartmann

The Grub Wrangler's Wisdom:

Chapter 11 Cooking Oils

    Out here on this vast horizon of cooking and baking, a whole herd of oils graze. Each with its own tale to tell, from its rich character to its detailed past. Here I've wrangled up a few of the most promising ones along with their details and a brief history. So let's tip our hats to them and take a gander at what they have to offer.

1. Olive Oil:
- Details: Olive oil is known for its fruity flavor and is rich in heart-healthy monounsaturated fats. It's often used in salad dressings, sautéing, and as a finishing oil.
- History: Olive oil has a rich history dating back thousands of years, especially in Mediterranean cultures. It was used not only in cooking but also for lighting lamps and for medicinal purposes.

2. Canola Oil:
- Details: Canola oil is light in flavor and has a high smoke point, making it versatile for cooking methods like frying and baking. It's low in saturated fat and high in monounsaturated fats.
- History: Canola oil originates from rapeseed oil but was developed in Canada (hence the name "canola") to create an oil low in erucic acid, which can be harmful. It became popular in the 1970s.

3. Coconut Oil:
- Details: Coconut oil has a distinct coconut flavor and is solid at room temperature. It's often used in baking and cooking in tropical cuisines.
- History: Coconut oil has a long history in tropical regions and has been used for cooking and skincare for centuries.

4. Vegetable Oil:
- Details: Vegetable oil is a generic term for various plant-based oils, including soybean, corn, and sunflower oil. They have neutral flavors and high smoke points.
- History: Vegetable oils became popular in the early 20th century due to advancements in food processing techniques, especially the extraction of oil from soybeans and corn.

Chrissy Hartmann

5. Ghee:
 - Details: Ghee is a form of clarified butter with a nutty flavor and a high smoke point. It's common in Indian cuisine and is used for sautéing and frying.
 - History: Ghee has been used in Indian cooking for centuries. It's a staple ingredient in many traditional dishes and is also considered sacred in some Indian rituals.

6. Avocado Oil:
 - Details: Avocado oil is a monounsaturated fat-rich oil with a mild flavor. It's often used in salad dressings, sautéing, and as a finishing oil.
 - History: Avocado oil has become more popular in recent years as avocados gained widespread popularity for their health benefits.

7. Palm Oil:
 - Details: Palm oil is commonly used in processed foods, but it has a higher saturated fat content. It is derived from the fruit of the oil palm tree.
 - History: Palm oil has been used for centuries in various parts of the world. Concerns about its environmental impact and health effects have led to increased scrutiny and efforts to source sustainable palm oil.

8. Sesame Oil:
 - Details: Sesame oil has a distinctive nutty flavor and is used in Asian cuisines for stir-frying, sautéing, and as a condiment.
 - History: Sesame oil has a long history in Asian and Middle Eastern cuisines. It's known for its rich flavor and aroma.

9. Peanut Oil:
 - Details: Peanut oil has a mild, nutty flavor and a high smoke point. It's often used in frying and for making peanut sauces.
 - History: Peanut oil is common in Asian and American cuisines. It's been used for deep-frying and cooking for decades.

10. Sunflower Oil:
 - Details: Sunflower oil is light in flavor and is suitable for various cooking methods. It's often used for frying and baking.
 - History: Sunflower oil is made from the seeds of the sunflower plant and has been widely used for cooking and frying in many countries.

11. Flaxseed Oil:
-Details: Flaxseed oil is celebrated for its omega-3 fatty acids and potential health benefits. Often taken as a dietary supplement to increase omega-3 intake, promote heart health, and reduce inflammation. Its nutty flavor makes it a great addition to vinaigrettes and dressings.
-History: Flaxseed oil, also known as linseed oil, has a long history of use. It was one of the first oils to be used for its drying properties in paintings and varnishes. In terms of culinary use, flaxseed oil gained prominence due to its high omega-3 fatty acid content, especially alpha-linolenic acid (ALA). It is considered a healthy oil due to its nutritional profile.
However, it should not be used for cooking due to its low smoke point, which can lead to the development of harmful compounds.

12. Hempseed Oil
- Details: Hemp oil is known for its nutty flavor and rich nutrient content. It is typically used for salad dressings as its distinct flavor makes it a great choice for vinaigrettes and dressings. Use it as a finishing oil over dishes like pasta or grilled vegetables. It can also be added to smoothies for an extra nutritional boost. Finally, hemp oil is used in some skincare products for its moisturizing and anti-inflammatory properties.
- History: Derived from the seeds of the hemp plant, a variety of Cannabis sativa. Hemp has a long history of use, both for its seeds and fibers. Hemp oil has gained popularity in recent years due to the growing interest in hemp-based products and the recognition of its potential health benefits.

13. Safflower Oil:
- Details: Safflower cultivation has spread to various regions worldwide. The oil is known for its high-smoke point making it suitable for frying and cooking at high temperatures without breaking down. It comes in two main varieties, high oleic and high linoleic. High oleic safflower oil is rich in monounsaturated fats offering potential health benefits. On the other hand, high linoleic safflower oil contains a higher proportion of polyunsaturated fats. Safflower oil is often praised for its mild versatility in cooking applications and its potential health benefits including being a source of mega 6 fatty acids; however, like any cooking oil, it is essential to use it in moderation and as part of a balanced diet.
- History: A vegetable oil extracted from the seeds of the safflower plant, carthamus tinctorius believed to have originated in ancient Egypt.

Now remember partner, each of these oils has a unique flavor, smoke point, and nutritional profile, making them fit for a roundup of different cooking and baking jobs. The choice of them there oils often depends on the specific grub you're rustling up, folks eating habits, and the flavors that are brought in from other parts of the country.

So, partner, there isn't no wrong trail when picking an oil. Just keep an eye on those smoke signals and flavors. You don't want them dinner guests looking at you like a bull in a China shop, do you?

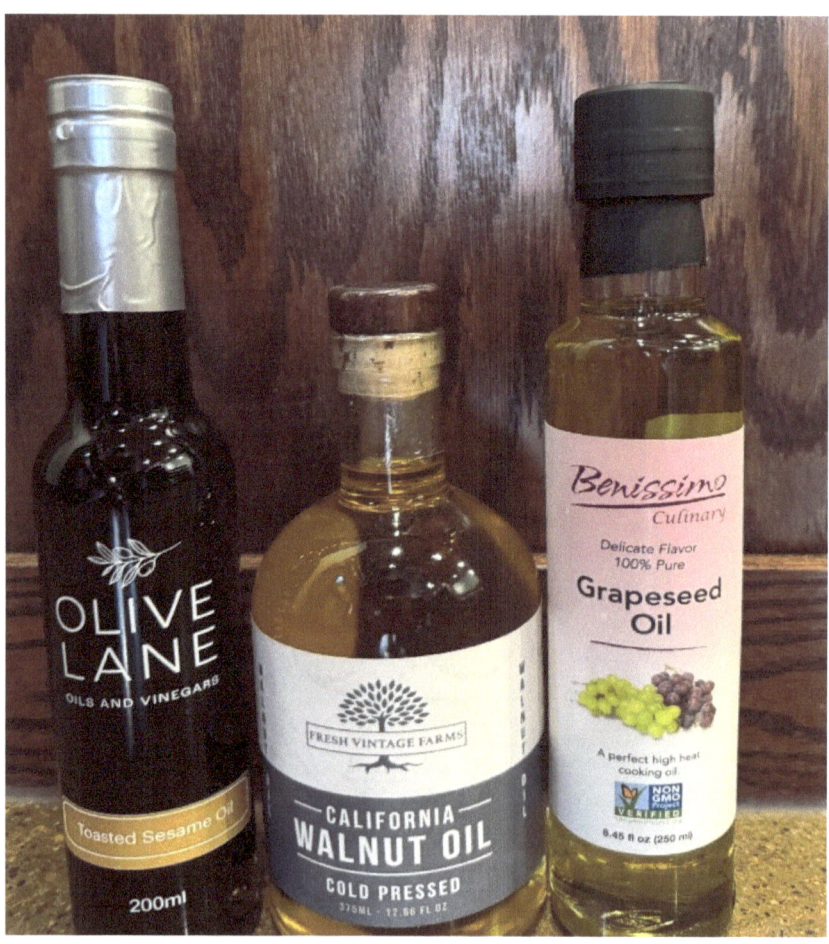

The Grub Wrangler's Wisdom:

Chrissy Hartmann

11.1 More On Vegetable Oils

Alright, cowboys, listen up, I know in the last section , we said it didn't matter what oil you fancied, but now let's mosey down the trail and delve a little deeper into the vegetable oils and what in tarnation qualifies as a vegetable oil.

You and I both know that vegetable oils have played a significant role in modern cooking, offering versatility, bang for your buck, and a shelf life longer than a coyote's howl. Their use has been shaped by the ways of the land, the March of technological progress, and the shifting winds of ever-changing taste. While them there veggie oils provide many advantages, it's essential to choose top -quality options and use them in moderation as part of a balanced diet.

These here veggie oils come straight from the heart of the land, drawn from a whole corral of plants and such. They are like the tried-and-true saddle in today's cooking and have a rich history. With a little digging, here's a tale about the nitty gritty on some of these here popular vegetable oils.

1. Soybean Oil:
- History: Soybean oil is a relatively recent addition to the cooking oil scene. It gained prominence in the mid-20th century, following advances in soybean farming and oil extraction. Today, it's one of the most widely produced and consumed vegetable oils globally.
- Details: Soybean oil has a neutral flavor, a high smoke point, and a balanced fatty acid profile. It is versatile, used in frying, baking, sautéing, and salad dressings.

2. Corn Oil:
- History: Corn oil has been in use for over a century but saw a surge in popularity in the mid-20th century due to the widespread cultivation of corn in the United States. It became a common household cooking oil.
- Details: Corn oil is another widely used vegetable oil known for its mild flavor and high smoke point. It contains a mix of polyunsaturated and monounsaturated fats. It is suitable for frying, baking, and general cooking.

3. Sunflower Oil:

- History: Sunflower oil, primarily produced from sunflower seeds, has been a traditional cooking oil in many parts of the world, especially in Eastern Europe and Russia. Its use spread to other regions as sunflower cultivation increased.
- Details: Sunflower oil comes from sunflower seeds and has a neutral flavor. It's light in color and has a high smoke point. It is versatile and is used for frying, sautéing, baking, and salad dressings.

4. Canola Oil:
- History: Canola oil originated from rapeseed oil but was developed in Canada in the 1970s to create an oil low in erucic acid, which can be harmful. The term "canola" stands for "Canadian oil, low acid." It was marketed as a healthy alternative to other oils.
- Details: Canola oil is low in saturated fat and has a neutral flavor. It's one of the healthiest vegetable oils and has a high smoke point. It is used for frying, baking, sautéing, and as a salad oil.

5. Palm Oil:
- History: Palm oil has a long history of use in regions where oil palm trees are native, particularly in West Africa and Southeast Asia. It has been used for cooking, skincare, and as an ingredient in various traditional dishes. However, the expansion of palm oil production has raised environmental and sustainability concerns.
- Details: Palm oil is derived from the fruit of oil palm trees. It is known for its red color and high saturated fat content. It is commonly used in processed foods and industrial applications. It's less common in home cooking.

Chrissy Hartmann

The Grub Wrangler's Wisdom:

11.2 Storage Life of Oils

Storing oils, be it any type of oil and yes that does include the various veggie oils, is crucial in keeping them top notch and safe for your chuckwagon cooking. Now let me spill the beans on how to stash them away and keeping them proper like and how long you can count on them staying good:

1. Grapeseed Oil:
-Storage: To prevent spoilage shield from oxygen, heat, and light. Keep lid tightly sealed.
- Shelf Life: Sealed 6 months, but once unsealed, the pantry shelf life is 3 months and if stored in the refrigerator it is 1 year, but unsealed it is 6 months.

2. Olive Oil:
- Storage: Store in a cool, dark place, away from direct sunlight and heat. Keep the bottle tightly sealed.
- Shelf Life: Extra virgin olive oil can last up to 2 years when stored properly, while other types of olive oil may have a longer shelf life.

3. Canola Oil:
- Storage: Store in a cool, dry place, and tightly close the bottle. Avoid exposing it to direct light.
- Shelf Life: Canola oil can last up to 1-2 years.

4. Sunflower Oil:
- Storage: Keep sunflower oil in a cool, dark place and ensure the container is sealed.
- Shelf Life: Sunflower oil typically has a shelf life of about 1 year.

5. Corn Oil:
- Storage: Store in a cool and dry location, and make sure the container is tightly sealed.
- Shelf Life: Corn oil can last for about 6-12 months.

6. Soybean Oil:
- Storage: Keep soybean oil in a cool, dark place, and ensure the container is tightly sealed.
- Shelf Life: Soybean oil generally has a shelf life of 6-12 months.

Chrissy Hartmann

7. Palm Oil:
- Storage: Store palm oil in a cool and dark place. It may solidify at lower temperatures, but that's normal. It can be kept at room temperature.
- Shelf Life: Palm oil can last for several months to a few years, depending on factors like purity and storage conditions.

8. Vegetable Oil Blends (e.g., vegetable oil):
- Storage: Similar to other oils, store in a cool, dark place with the container tightly sealed.
- Shelf Life: Vegetable oil blends typically have a shelf life of 6-12 months.

9. Hempseed Oil:
-Storage: To maintain the quality of hemp oil Store it in the refrigerator to prevent rancidity and preserve its nutritional value. Ensure the container is tightly sealed.
- Shelf Life: Use it within a few weeks to a few months after opening to ensure freshness.

10. Flaxseed Oil:
- Storage: To maintain the quality of flaxseed oil keep it in the refrigerator to slow down the oxidation process. Use dark-colored glass containers to protect it from light.
- Shelf Life: Consume it within a few weeks to a few months after opening to ensure freshness.

11. Safflower Oil
- Storage: For monounsaturated keep it in a cool, dark place, such as a cupboard. For the polyunsaturated should be stored in the refrigerator.
- Shelf Life: Monounsaturated and polyunsaturated for up to six months.

Alrighty, partner, with all them tidbits, we don't reckon you should overlook it. those oils got a shelf life that varies on factors like the oil's purity, exposure to light and heat, and the quality of the oil when first bought. So, remember this, it won't do you and your ticker no good, if you don't choose wisely. So, pick an oil like you'd picking a trusty steed, cowboy.

11.3 Signs of Rancid Oils

From one chuckwagon cook to another, there are those times, the oils just go plumb bad. Here are the signs that I've included that signal an oil has gone rancid:

- a sour or off odor
- a noticeable change in taste.

If you notice these signs, it's best to discard the oil.

To extend the shelf life of your cooking oils, you can also consider refrigeration, especially for oils like flaxseed or hempseed oil, which are more prone to spoilage due to their high polyunsaturated fat content. Additionally, using clean, dry utensils to scoop oil from the container and avoiding cross-contamination can lend a hand to maintain oil quality.

Chrissy Hartmann

The Grub Wrangler's Wisdom:

11.4 Types of Fats Found in Cooking Oils

    Okay, cowboy, I reckon you know this by now, but here's a refresher. There are three main types of fats found in cooking oils:
- saturated fats
- unsaturated fats (monounsaturated and polyunsaturated)
- trans fats.

The Types of Fats
1. Saturated Fats:
- Benefits: Provides stability for cooking at high temperatures.
- Dangers: Excessive intake may contribute to elevated cholesterol levels.
- Oils: Coconut oil, palm oil.

2. Monounsaturated Fats:
- Benefits: Can have heart health benefits.
- Dangers: High calorie content; moderation is key.
- Oils: Olive oil and Canola oil.

3. Polyunsaturated Fats:
- Benefits: Essential fatty acids, including omega-3 and omega-6.
- Dangers: Susceptible to oxidation; balance is important.
- Oils: grapeseed oil, soybean oil, corn oil, and sunflower oil.

4. Trans Fats:
- Benefits: No inherent health benefits.
- Dangers: Increases bad cholesterol, lowers good cholesterol.
- Oils: Partially hydrogenated oils (artificial trans fats) found in some processed foods; many countries have banned or restricted their use.

    *Choosing oils with a balance of these fats and being mindful of overall fat intake, contributes to a ticker-healthy diet. Grapeseed oil is primarily composed of polyunsaturated fats, particularly omega-6 fatty acids. It's low in saturated fat and has a moderate amount of monounsaturated fat.

Chrissy Hartmann

The breakdown:

Polyunsaturated Fats:
- High Amount: About 70% (mainly omega-6)
- Benefits: Essential fatty acids, including linoleic acid.

: Monounsaturated Fats:
- Moderate amount: About 20%
- Benefits: Provides additional cardiovascular benefits.

Saturated Fats:
- Low amount: About 10%.
- Benefits: Suitable for cooking at moderate temperatures.

    Grapeseed oil is often praised for its mild flavor and high smoke point, making it suitable for various cooking methods. While it offers some health benefits for the ticker, your taste buds, and aids in preventing the inflammation of your cells , it's essential to maintain a balanced intake of the different good fats for optimal health.

The Grub Wrangler's Wisdom:

Chrissy Hartmann

Chapter 12 Culinary Techniques

Here's the spread on detailed directions for various culinary techniques along with some grub examples for good measure:

1. Roasting:
- Directions: Preheat your oven to the desired temperature (usually around 375-420°F. Place the ingredient on a baking sheet, drizzle with oil, season with salt and pepper, and roast until it's tender and slightly caramelized.
- Food Example: Roasting asparagus with grapeseed oil, salt, and pepper until it's tender and has crispy edges.

2. Sautéing:
- Directions: Heat a pan over medium-high heat, add oil, and let it get hot. Add the ingredient and stir or toss it frequently in the hot oil until it's browned and cooked through.
- Food Example: Sautéing diced onions in grapeseed oil until they become translucent and slightly golden.

3. Mincing:
- Directions: Use a sharp knife to cut the ingredient into very fine pieces, almost to the point of turning it into a paste.
- Food Example: Mincing garlic into tiny pieces to incorporate it evenly into a sauce.

4. Dicing:
- Directions: Cut the ingredient into uniformly sized small cubes, typically around 1/4 to 1/2 inch in size.
- Food Example: Dicing tomatoes for a fresh salsa.

5. Chopping:
- Directions: Cut the ingredient into larger, irregular pieces. The size can vary depending on your preference.
- Food Example: Chopping bell peppers into pieces for a stir-fry.

6. Grating/Zesting:
- Directions: Use a grater or zester to scrape against the grater to create fine shreds or zest from the ingredient's outer peel.

- Food Example: Grating cheese for a pasta dish or zesting lemon for a lemon-infused dressing.

These techniques are fundamental in cooking and can be put to work on a wide spread of ingredients for creating various dishes. Now here in Texas, we love it big. In fact, the bigger the better, but let's not go hog wild. Because as sure as the stars come out at night, the size and method you choose depend on the recipe's requirements and your cowboys desired texture and flavor. So, use some caution here and take notes on what works best for your chuckwagon.

Chrissy Hartmann

The Grub Wrangler's Wisdom:

Chapter 13 Cooking Conversions

When you're rustling up grub in the chuckwagon, keep an eye on those measurements and temperatures. Whether your trading teaspoons for tablespoons or figuring out how hot the Dutch oven needs to be, it's crucial to know Fahrenheit to Celsius and cups to gallons, mastering the conversions ensures your cooking is spot on. So, saddle up and wrangle them numbers, partner, cause a well-cooked trail feast is the key to a happy cowboy.

Chrissy Hartmann

13.1 Measurement Conversions

3 teaspoons = 1 Tablespoon
1 tablespoon = 1/16 cup
2 tablespoons = 1/8 cup
4 tablespoons = 1/4 cup
5 tablespoons and one teaspoon = 1/3 cup
8 tablespoons = 1/2 cup
12 tablespoons = 3/4 cups
16 tablespoons = 1 cup

2 ounces = 1/8 pound
4 ounces = 1/4 pound
8 ounces = 1/2 pounds
16 ounces = 1 pound

1 tablespoon = 1/2 fluid ounces
2 tablespoons = 1 fluid ounce
4 tablespoons = 2 fluid ounces
6 tablespoons = 3 fluid ounces
8 tablespoons = 4 fluid ounces

1 cup = one-half pint
2 cups = one pint
2 pints = 1 quart
4 quarts = 1 gallon

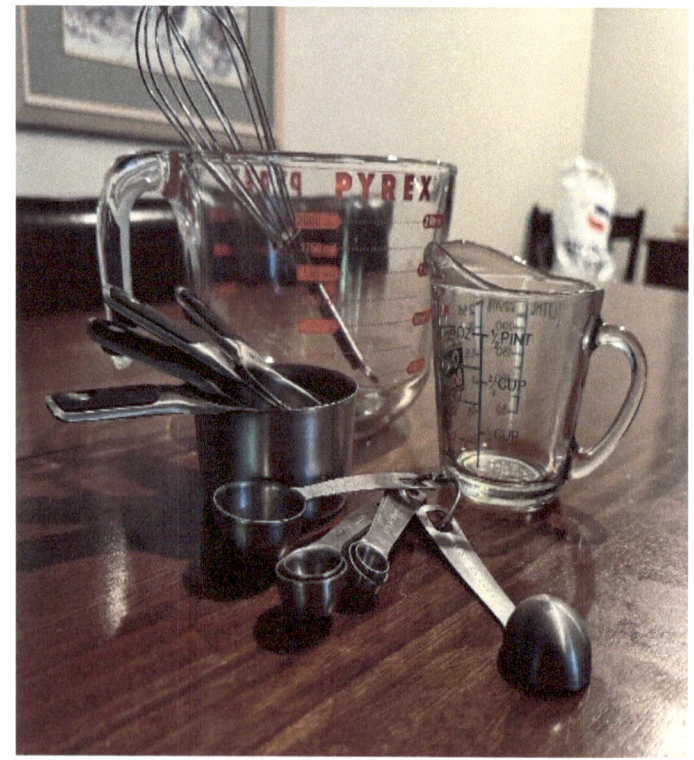

13.2 Temperature Conversions

Fahrenheit (°F) = Celsius (°C)

250°F = 121°C
275°F = 135°C
300°F = 149°C
325°F = 163°C
350°F = 177°C
375°F = 191°C
400°F = 204°C
425°F = 218°C
450°F = 232°C
475°F = 246°C
500°F = 260°C

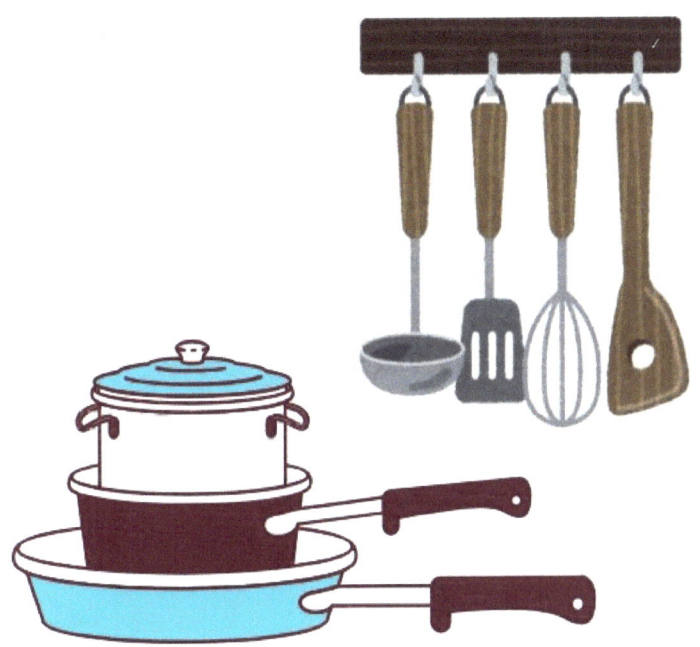

Chrissy Hartmann

13.3 Target Temperatures

In the wild, a cowboy might risk a tumble with a wild stallion, but when it comes to cooking meat, there's no room for wild gambles. Cooking your meat to the right temperature isn't just a culinary ritual; it's the sheriff in the town of food safety, ensuring your taste buds enjoy the rodeo without a stampede of bacteria ruining the show.

Now, picture this: you're out on the range, rustling up a hearty steak. Just like you wouldn't ride a bronco blindfolded, you shouldn't cook meat without knowing it's reached the safe haven of proper temperature. The stakes are high – too low, and you're dancing with uninvited guests like salmonella or E. coli. Too high, and your steak turns into a leather saddle. We're aiming for that sweet spot where the flavors are tender, and the pathogens are left in the dust.

So, partner, grab your trusty food thermometer, the six-shooter of the culinary world and make sure that beef, pork, poultry, and fish hit their target temperatures. It's not just about winning the showdown against undercooked meat; it's about saving yourself from a stomach tumble that even the toughest cowboy wouldn't ride willingly. Stick to the rules of the west , and your taste buds will be tip-tapping like a boot scooting boogie at a barn dance.

Cook safe, eat hearty, and may your steaks be as rare as a desert oasis at high noon. Safe minimum internal temperatures for various meats are crucial to ensure they're properly cooked and safe to eat. The recommended minimum internal temperatures for different meats for various cooking methods are:

1. Beef, Pork, Lamb, and Veal:
- Steaks and Roasts: 145°F (63°C)
- Ground Meats: 160°F (71°C)

2. Chicken and Turkey:
- Breasts, Roasts, and Thighs: 165°F (74°C)
- Ground Chicken or Turkey: 165°F (74°C)

3. Fish:
- Whole Fish: 145°F (63°C)

- Fish Fillets: 145°F (63°C)

4. Shrimp:
- Cook until opaque and firm; internal temperature may not be as relevant. About 2 minutes each side.

In general, always use a food thermometer to check the internal temperature at the thickest part of the meat to ensure it reaches the safe minimum temperature.

Chrissy Hartmann

Grub Wrangler's Wisdom:

Chapter 14 Cowboy-style Glossary

Howdy, culinary wanderers! Welcome to the roundup of flavors and techniques that'll have you cooking like a seasoned trail chef. In this here glossary, we've corralled a posse of cowboy phrases to guide you through the wild terrain of the kitchen. From whisking up frothy eggs that'd make a mustang jealous to braising meat as tender as a mother's touch, these expressions will be your trusty companions on the culinary trail. So, don your apron, saddle up your spatula, and let's mosey through this cookbook hoedown, where the spirit of the west meets the sizzle of the skillet. And just think, you might one day sound like your favorite chuckwagon cook. Yeehaw!
Happy cooking, partners!

1. Sifting the flour to resemble desert sand: Preparing dry ingredients with care so it blends in evenly.
2. Simmering low and slow like a cattle drive: Cooking a dish at a gentle temperature for rich flavors.
3. Wrangling up the perfect spice roundup: Crafting a well-balanced blend of seasonings.
4. Flipping flapjacks with a flick of the wrist: Mastering the art of pancake perfection.
5. Sharpening knives like honing a cowboy's blade: Ensuring your cutlery is ready for the culinary showdown.
6. Riding the gravy train: Creating a luscious sauce to complement your grub.
7. Letting the dough rise like a morning sun: Allowing bread to proof and swell to perfection.
8. Searing steaks hotter than a branding iron: Achieving a golden crust for a juicy steak.
9. Whipping up a storm in the mixing bowl: Creating a flurry of flavors in a well-blended concoction.
10. Chopping veggies finer than a cattle brand: Precisely preparing vegetables for a delightful dish.
11. Measuring with the precision of a surveyor: Ensuring accurate quantities for the perfect recipe.
12. Sauteing onions till they sing like a campfire tune: Cooking onions until they reach a sweet, caramelized melody.
13. Baking biscuits golden as the prairie sun: Achieving that ideal biscuit color and texture.
14. Smoking and roasting like a seasoned trail cook: Mastering the art of smoking and roasting meats.

Chrissy Hartmann

15. Folding in ingredients with the grace of a dance partner: Combining elements gently for a harmonious dish.
16. Making gravy from scratch, not from a can: Crafting a homemade gravy that's pure cowboy comfort.
17. Building layers like a bunkhouse bed: Creating intricate, flavorful layers in casseroles or desserts.
18. Brewing coffee stronger than a rancher's handshake: Preparing a robust cup of cowboy coffee.
19. Toasting nuts like a campfire tale: Enhancing the flavor of nuts through careful toasting.
20. Garnishing with flair, like branding cattle with style: Adding a finishing touch to your dish with finesse.
21. Rolling out pie crusts flatter than the horizon: Achieving the perfect thickness for a delectable pie.
22. Seasoning cast iron with the patience of a cattle drive: Building a well-seasoned and reliable cast-iron skillet.
23. Sharing secrets of marinades that sing like a cowboy ballad: Infusing meats with flavors that harmonize like a Western melody.
24. Cracking eggs smoother than a bronco ride: Mastering the art of egg-cracking for a seamless culinary experience.
25. Braising meat tender as a mother's touch: Slow-cooking meat until it's tender and full of love.
26. Making a roux thicker than a buffalo hide: Creating a rich, hearty base for sauces and gravies.
27. Whisking up frothy eggs like a lathered-up mustang: Achieving the perfect consistency in beaten eggs.
28. Smoking your BBQ like a prairie wildfire: Infusing meats with that irresistible smoky flavor.
29. Bringing meat sweeter than a cowboy's dream: Enhancing meat with a flavorful brine for maximum juiciness.
30. Dressing salads crisper than autumn leaves: Preparing salads with fresh and crisp ingredients.
31. Mixing cocktails with the finesse of a saloon barkeep: Crafting beverages that dance on the taste buds.
32. Stirring pots deeper than a prospector's dig: Ensuring even cooking and melding of flavors in your pot.

33. Dropping biscuits on the sheet like rain on a tin roof: Placing biscuits evenly for a perfect bake.
34. Crafting marinades with the boldness of a cattle brand: Creating flavorful concoctions to elevate your meats.
35. Measuring like a trailblazer with a keen eye for detail: Guaranteeing precise measurements for culinary success.
36. Baking cornbread golden as a harvest moon: Achieving that golden hue for the perfect cornbread.
37. Roasting vegetables tender as a prairie breeze: Bringing out the best in veggies with a roasting touch.
38. Making vinaigrettes lighter than a tumbleweed's roll: Preparing dressings that add a refreshing zing to salads.
39. Kneading dough with the patience of a shepherd with his flock: Ensuring the right consistency and texture in your dough.
40. Plating dishes with the artistry of a Western sunset: Presenting your culinary creations with a touch of flair and elegance.
41. The Grub Wrangler's Wisdom: Recipe notes of this here current chuckwagon cook.

Chrissy Hartmann

The Grub Wrangler's Wisdom:

Dear Reader:

Thanks for taking a gander at my first ever cookbook. I honestly hope you enjoy using it as much as I did creating it. It's been like a twister on the plains creating and photographing these here recipes and putting together this book. Believe it or not, but grapeseed oil is the true blessing in my life and is probably one of the reason's I'm still here and not laying out on Boot Hill six feet under.

I hope you find as much success with your health that I have with using this oil. My only regret is that I didn't start using it sooner.

If you have time, let me know what you think with a review on Amazon or Good Reads. And don't ever hesitate to contact me regarding any questions on grapeseed oil, because I'd be sure happy and tickled pink to try and assist.

If you have any questions, thoughts, praise, or complaints please send me an e-mail to my publisher who hog ties me to her desk while she reads all my mail to me.

Send up a smoke signal to me at
prickleforrestllc@sssnet.com

Thanks,

Chrissy Hartmann

Chrissy Hartmann

Chrissy's Other Books……

Chrissy's other books can be found on her website, https://ChrissyHartmann.com/books with links to purchase worldwide.

Check out:

Rescuing Whiskey's Salvation
A 5 star Readers Favorite

Cherishing Whiskey's Salvation

And
 Her short story that kicks off a new group of short stories regarding the Whiskey Salvation series
Love on the Lakefront: Romantic Tales from the Great Lakes
With Chrissy's short story:
Tacking of Hearts

 Follow Chrissy on social media at USAWriter355 to get more information.

About The Author…

Not one to let the crack of dawn start the day without her and someone who burns the midnight oil staying up long enough to tuck in the moon and stars, Chrissy Hartmann can be found writing novels, polishing her latest short story, and/or even posting her freshly pressed blog.

Creating is always on the brain whether it be writing, concocting a new recipe for possibly another cookbook, or even designing shoes for her garden geese. She's not one to let time idle away, not in less she has a good book and a strong cup of coffee. Her family keeps her on the go with spinning vinyl or galloping off to explore a quaint small town or two.

At present, with the completion of her cookbook, The Grub Wrangler: Heartfelt Grapeseed Oil Recipes with Benefits," she's also published her first novella, Cherishing Whiskey's Salvation that goes along with her debut novel, Rescuing Whiskey's Salvation. Now she's back to working on her third novel to the Whiskey Salvation Series, Treasuring Whiskey's Salvation and polishing up her anthology of short stories, Tales from The Prickle Forrest, which is planned for release in 2025.

Plus let's not forget about her newest novella, a Christmas story for the Whiskey Salvation series, Twelve Days of Christmas Deeds," arriving late fall of 2024.

All books including this here cookbook will be available through Amazon, Ingram , Google Play, Barnes and Noble, Apple, and Books2Read. And autographed copies are available on her website to at https://chrissyhartmann.com/shop

You can visit her on X, Truth Social, Facebook, and Instagram @USAWriter355 or check out her website https://chrissyhartmann.com/

More on this cowgirl can be acquired if you join her newsletter the Prickle Forrest Chronicles at https://PrickleForrestChronicles.com/follow-me

 job as editor in chief of Prickle Forrest Books where she'll be leading the charge on author interviews, sensitivity critiques, book reviews, and developmental edits. She can be found here:
https://PrickleForrestBooks.com/

And speaking of book reviews, Chrissy loves to get them for her own books. The ones who have really enjoyed her books, tickle her heart. And those that give her a few negative prickles, well, they just help to spur her on to better writing. She appreciates the honesty. And even though she may not get a 5-star review from you, she does appreciate your time to read her work. Please leave a review at
Good Reads, Amazon, and any online retailer of your choice. Thanks!

Chrissy Hartmann

Index

Introduction and Background
- Introduction 1
- History of Grapeseed oil 3
- Culinary Benefits 4
- Grapeseed Oil Health Benefits 5
- Dangers of Grapeseed Oil 7
- The Making of Grapeseed Oil 9
- Grapeseed Oil Production 10
- Grapeseed Oil vs. Grapeseed Extract 11
- Grape Varieties and Grapeseed Production 12–14
- Reasons for Choosing Grapeseed Oil 15
- Grapeseed Antioxidants 16
- Grape Varieties 18
- Nutritional Value and Daily Allowances 20–21
- Grapeseed Oil – Safe for the trail if Ridden Right 22

Appetizers
- Buckshot Brussel Sprouts 108
- Butternut Chipotle Turkey Chili 46
- Cauliflower Cow Patties 62
- Chicken Pepper Cranberry Salad 54
- Chipotle Chicken Wings 63
- Cowboy Salad 90
- Crispy Chipotle Kale Chips 110
- Fire Blackened Shrimp 56
- Grilled Veggie Bob 53
- Mediterranean Lemon Salad 97
- Pony Up Pasta Salad 107
- Plum Delicious Fried Greenies 60
- Robust Spinach Artichoke Dip 48
- Rustic Chili Potato Wedges 52
- Smokey Orange Cauliflower Wings 50
- Spicy Hummus with Fresh Veggies 44

Blackened
- Blackened Catfish with Lemon Cream Sauce   66
- Fire Blackened Shrimp   56

Beef
- Chipotle Steak Taco   77
- Rodeo Peppered Beef   76
- Rustler's Beef Stew   80
- Spirited Beef Stir-Fry   70

Breads
- Chuckwagon Cornbread   112
- Pumpkin Harvest Berry Bread   40
- Texas Sunshine Muffins   38
- Trails End Banana Bread   122
- Western Banana-Cran Bites   32

Breakfast
- Blueberry Flapjacks   26
- Cowboy Granola Crunch   33
- Healthy Morning Smoothie   28
- Saddle Hearty Oatmeal   30
- Western Banana-Cran Bites   32
- Western Sunrise Slices   29

Breakfast Drinks
- Healthy Morning Smoothie   28

Cakes
- Apple Cinnamon Cake   124
- Colorado Berry Crumble   120
- Homestead Pumpkin Funnel Cakes   132
- Iowa Dusty Delights   118
- Lemon Herding Cakes   130
- Texas Carrot Cake   136

Chipotle
- Butternut Chipotle Turkey Chili   46
- Chipotle Chicken Wings   63

Chrissy Hartmann

- Chipotle Shrimp Scampi   69
- Chipotle Steak Taco   77
- Crispy Chipotle Kale Chips   110

Cookies
- Cowboy Cookies   138
- Cowboy Cow Chips   126

Delicious Desserts   117
- Apple Cinnamon Cake   124
- Colorado Berry Crumble   120
- Cowboy Cookies   138
- Cowboy Cow Chips   126
- Heavenly Berry Parfait   128
- Homestead Pumpkin Funnel Cakes   132
- Iowa Dusty Delights   118
- Lemon Herding Cakes   130
- Peanut Brittle   134
- Texas Carrot Cake   136
- Toasted Pecan Clusters   129
- Trails End Banana Bread   122

Dressings, Drizzles, and More   141
- Chipotle Drizzle   151
- Classic Balsamic Vinaigrette   142
- Honey Barbecue Sauce   152
- Honey Mustard Glaze   148
- Homemade Mayonnaise   150
- Lemon Cream Sauce   154
- Lemon-Honey Dijon Dressing   143
- Maple-Dijon Glaze   147
- Plum Delicious Ginger Dipping Sauce   155
- Raspberry-Lime Vinaigrette   146
- Sesame Dressing   144
- Spicy Vidalia Sauce   153
- Sweet-N-Sour Dressing   149
- Sweet Orange Dressing   145

Egg Dishes
- Feta Fiesta Spinach Eggs   36
- Texas Steak and Egg Fajita   35

Fruits
Apple
- Apple Cinnamon Cake   124
- Pork Tenderloin with Apple Compote   74

Banana
- Trails End Banana Bread   122
- Western Banana-Cran Bites   32

Berry
- Colorado Berry Crumble   120
- Healthy Morning Smoothie   28
- Heavenly Berry Parfait   128
- Pecan Berry Chicken   73
- Pumpkin Harvest Berry Bread   40

Cranberry
- Chicken Pepper Cranberry Salad   54
- Western Banana-Cran Bites   32

Lemon
- Blackened Catfish with Lemon Cream Sauce   66
- Lemon Broccoli   105
- Lemon Cream Sauce   154
- Lemon Herding Cakes   130
- Lemon-Honey Dijon Dressing   143
- Mediterranean Lemon Salad   97
- Zesty Lemon Chicken   68

Lime
- Raspberry-Lime Vinaigrette   146

Orange
- Smokey Orange Cauliflower Wings   50
- Sweet Orange Dressing   145

Chrissy Hartmann

Plum
- Plum Delicious Fried Greenies 60
- Plum Delicious Ginger Dipping Sauce 155

Pumpkin
- Homestead Pumpkin Funnel Cakes 132
- Pumpkin Harvest Berry Bread 40

Raspberry
- Raspberry-Lime Vinaigrette 146

Main Course Marvels 65
- Blackened Catfish with Lemon Cream Sauce 66
- Calico Beans 92
- Chicken Soft Taco 82
- Chipotle Shrimp Scampi 69
- Chipotle Steak Taco 77
- Christmas Spinach Chicken 75
- Cowboy Salad 90
- Pecan Berry Chicken 73
- Pork Tenderloin with Apple Compote 74
- Rodeo Peppered Beef 76
- Rustler's Beef Stew 80
- Seared Salmon 88
- Spirited Beef Stir-Fry 70
- Southwest Black Bean Burger 89
- Stuffed Sausage Peppers 84
- Sundance Tuna Melts 78
- Texas-Two Step Barbecue Chicken 86
- Woodland Mushroom Risotto 72
- Zesty Lemon Chicken 68

Nuts
- Peanut Brittle 134
- Pecan Berry Chicken 73
- Toasted Pecan Clusters 129

Pork
- Pork Tenderloin with Apple Compote   74
- Stuffed Sausage Peppers   84

Poultry
- Chipotle Chicken Wings   63
- Christmas Spinach Chicken   75
- Pecan Berry Chicken   73
- Turkey Stuffed Mushrooms   58
- Texas-Two Step Barbecue Chicken   86
- Zesty Lemon Chicken   68

Salads
- Chicken Pepper Cranberry Salad   54
- Cowboy Salad   90
- Lonestar Tater Salad   104
- Mediterranean Lemon Salad   97
- Pony Up Pasta Salad   107

Savory Starters   43
- Butternut Chipotle Turkey Chili   46
- Cauliflower Cow Patties   62
- Chicken Pepper Cranberry Salad   54
- Chipotle Chicken Wings   63
- Fire Blackened Shrimp   56
- Grilled Veggie Bob   53
- Plum Delicious Fried Greenies   60
- Robust Spinach Artichoke Dip   48
- Rustic Chili Potato Wedges   52
- Smokey Orange Cauliflower Wings   50
- Spicy Hummus with Fresh Veggies   44

Seafood
- Blackened Catfish with Lemon Cream Sauce   66
- Chipotle Shrimp Scampi   69
- Fire Blackened Shrimp   56
- Seared Salmon   88

Chrissy Hartmann

Satisfying Sidekicks 95
- Balsamic Glazed Carrots 102
- Buckshot Brussel Sprouts 108
- Campfire Roasted Asparagus 100
- Chuckwagon Cornbread 112
- Crispy Chipotle Kale Chips 110
- Green Bean Roundup with Bacon 99
- Lemon Broccoli 106
- Lonestar Tater Salad 105
- Mediterranean Lemon Salad 97
- Mushroom Onion Spinach Saute 98
- Pony Up Pasta Salad 108
- Spicy Sweet Taters 107
- Texas Hash 114
- Yukon Golden Roasted Potatoes 96

Snacks
- Crispy Chipotle Kale Chips 110
- Iowa Dusty Delights 118
- Western Banana-Cran Bites 32

Soups
- Butternut Chipotle Turkey Chili 46
- Woodland Mushroom Risotto 72

Steak
- Chipotle Steak Taco 77
- Texas Steak and Egg Fajita 35

Sunrise Delights 25
- Blueberry Flapjacks 26
- Cowboy Granola Crunch 33
- Feta Fiesta Spinach Eggs 36
- Healthy Morning Smoothie 28
- Pumpkin Harvest Berry Bread 40
- Saddle Hearty Oatmeal 30
- Texas Steak and Egg Fajita 35
- Texas Sunshine Muffins 38

- Western Banana-Cran Bites   32
- Western Sunrise Slices   29

Tacos and Fajitas
- Chicken Soft Taco   82
- Chipotle Steak Taco   78
- Texas Steak and Egg Fajita   35

Vegetables
Artichokes
- Robust Spinach Artichoke Dip   48

Asparagus
- Campfire Roasted Asparagus   100

Broccoli
- Lemon Broccoli   105

Brussel Sprouts
- Buckshot Brussel Sprouts   108

Butternut Squash
- Butternut Chipotle Turkey Chili   46

Cauliflower
- Cauliflower Cow Patties   62
- Smokey Orange Cauliflower Wings   50

Carrots
- Balsamic Glazed Carrots   102
- Texas Carrot Cake   136

Green Beans
- Green Bean Roundup with Bacon   99
- Plum Delicious Fried Greenies   60

Kale
- Crispy Chipotle Kale Chips   110

Chrissy Hartmann

Mushrooms
- Mushroom Onion Spinach Saute   98
- Turkey Stuffed Mushrooms   58
- Woodland Mushroom Risotto   72

Onions
- Mushroom Onion Spinach Saute   98

Peppers
- Stuffed Sausage Peppers   84

Potatoes
- Lonestar Tater Salad   105
- Rustic Chili Potato Wedges   52
- Spicy Sweet Taters   106
- Yukon Golden Roasted Potatoes   96

Spinach
- Christmas Spinach Chicken   75
- Feta Fiesta Spinach Eggs   36
- Mushroom Onion Spinach Saute   98
- Robust Spinach Artichoke Dip   48

Veggies
- Grilled Veggie Bob   53
- Spicy Hummus with Fresh Veggies   44

Cooking Techniques and Tips
- Baking Tips   159
- Cooking Tips   158
- Culinary Techniques   176
- Measurement Conversions   180
- Target Temperatures   182
- Temperature Conversions   181

Cooking Oils and Nutrition
- Cooking Oils Overview   161
- More on vegetable Oils   166

- Storage Life of Oils   169
- Rancid Oils   171
- Types of Fats in Cooking Oils   173

Glossary and Extras
- Cowboy-Style Glossary   185
- Dear Reader   189
- Chrissy's Other Books   190
- About the Author   191
- Index   192

Chrissy Hartmann